THE HORMONE MAKEOVER

7 Steps to Transform Your Life with Bioidentical Hormones

Donna White

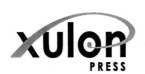

PRESS

contained in this book should be used to replace established, conventional medical approaches, especially in cases of emergencies, serious or life-threatening diseases or conditions. No information in this book should be used to replace conventional medical treatment or standard of care. Although the author and publisher have made every effort to ensure the accuracy and completeness of information contained in this book, we assume no responsibility for error, inaccuracies, omissions, or any inconsistency herein. Any slights of people, places or organizations are unintentional.

www.xulonpress.com

THE HORMONE MAKEOVER

7 Steps to Transform Your Life with Bioidentical Hormones

"I have had the opportunity to watch Donna's work develop over the last 8 years. I witnessed the program's success first hand as I worked with her when she started the program. I was and continue to be amazed at the outcomes. Donna is one of the most knowledgeable and personable experts I know in the area of bioidentical hormones."
Julius Torelli, MD FACC
High Point, NC

"Having worked with Donna for over two years I have seen the immensely positive effect her hormonal approach has had in transforming the lives of countless hundreds of patients. She has been able to effectively apply her vast knowledge in a way that makes "The Hormone Makeover" adaptable to each individual, reflecting the true art of medicine at its finest."
Larry Webster, MD

"Through Christian voice, research, personal experience and extensive clinical experience, Donna White triumphs. This book is very informative about the body's lifelong hormonal journey and how to safely maintain its balance via bioidentical hormone replacement therapy."
K. Andre' Sloan, RPh, MBA President,
Carolina Compounding & Nutritional Pharmacy (CCNP)
www.ccnprx.com

"This is a must have guide for all practitioners and any person interested in Bioidentical Hormones. The author has provided extensive clinical data and research in this condensed reference book that is sure to enlighten all readers!"
Kristen Spratt, MSN, FNP Dr Kanelos, Carolina Family Healthcare Ballentyne

"In today's world of conflicting messages from the medical community, clarity is in demand. I have known Donna White for five years and the message and education she delivers has changed the lives of many through her passion for helping women achieve natural hormone balance. Finally there is some real clarity from her insightful work that will encourage and educate women who are struggling to get back to their true selves. I applaud Donna for not only providing us the knowledge needed but also for allowing her faith in God to lead her way."
Matt Monroe
President & Founder
PEOPLESWAY

"Donna White demystifies the world of female hormones, while bringing hope to women who suffer from hormonal imbalance in her informative, user friendly book."
Kimber Britner
Speaker, Author, Coach
www.ignitinghearts.com

"When you have experienced first hand most of the symptoms that Donna describes in her book as I have; you will appreciate all of the research and experience that goes into the pages of this much needed book. It has certainly paid off for she has definitely outdone herself in the extensive information on bio-identical hormones and synthetic hormones. Donna backs up with facts in this book what she has been telling women all over the USA for years. Understanding the symptoms is so important but having a way to test hormones to

find out what is going on in our bodies and then being able to take the hormone(s) that our body needs to make us ''sane'' again is a real blessing. The Hormone Makeover is written in such a way that it is easy to understand by anyone. Every women should have a copy to use as a helps book when they need info on the things that are going on in their bodies hormonally. Thanks to Donna my husband now recognizes the woman that he wakes up to in the morning and no longer wonders what happened to his loving wife. Women need this information and finally it is here in The Hormone Makeover.''
Pastor Judy Harmon
Ultimate Life Church
www.ultimatelifeministries.com

ACKNOWLEDGMENTS

I would like to acknowledge and thank my husband, Jack, for helping make my dreams come true. You are the most wonderful husband in the world. Thank you for understanding my hormones. My children and family are the loves of my life.

I would like to dedicate this book to women dealing with hormonal challenges, your families, your destinies and all that pertains to your lives. May you face each day with balanced hormones and abundant health. Be encouraged, educated and equipped in regard to your health and hormones by this book.

TABLE OF CONTENTS

Foreword

Signature Wellness,
Ballantyne **Introduction**

Chapter 1

Chapter 2

Chapter 3

Chapter 4

Chapter 5

FOREWORD

If you have picked up this book and wonder if you might need a Hormone Makeover, let me explain why you might just be right!

Your body is complex, with various intertwining systems. Although medicine has often thought of the various systems as separate, in truth they function in harmony. If one or more hormones should become out of "balance", this can have an impact on other hormones, with far reaching effects in many different systems.

In this book, Donna White carefully lays out the interconnectedness of our hormonal system. She explains how different hormones can influence our nervous system, immune system, digestive system, cardiovascular system, reproductive system and how hormones affect virtually all of the important functions of the body. Different hormone imbalances contribute to different problems; practical information is provided to help you understand how hormones may be contributing to your symptoms.

Answers are provided to many important questions: What are hormones? What is the difference between bioidentical and synthetic hormones? Could your symptoms be a result of a hormone imbalance? Background science is provided to show that all hormone therapies are NOT equal. Armed with this knowledge, women will be equipped with the know-how to make well-informed decisions they can feel confident about.

Every individual has a unique hormonal makeup, and our bodies have different needs for different hormones at different times of our lives. This book carefully explains the need for working in a partnership with a knowledgeable healthcare provider to customize your treatment so that it is exactly right for you.

Donna White has been helping women to balance their hormones for over a decade, and I am privileged to have the opportunity to work with her. She is an excellent teacher – both to her patients, helping them to understand their complex hormonal puzzle, and to the many health care professionals she has helped to train over the years. She understands that hormones are not a sole magical panacea and that a holistic approach to wellness is necessary. She cares about helping women, and that dedication shows in her work.

Please read this book and use this information to guide your discussion with your healthcare provider. A Hormone Makeover may be just what you need to feel like yourself again!

Deborah Matthew, MD
Fellowship trained and Board Certified in Anti-Aging,
Regenerative and Functional Medicine by the American Academy of Anti-Aging Medicine
Founder and Medical Director, Signature Wellness Center for Optimal Health

INTRODUCTION

I would like to start by sharing my heart with you. First of all, I have known for years that I was to write a book about hormones for women. When that long-awaited season arrived, doubts set in. Can you relate? There are so many books about hormones on the market already. Why should I write yet another one? That gentle, small voice in my spirit seemed to say, "Yes, but you are to write one specifically to *My* women." At that moment, it all made perfect sense. You see, for the past fifteen years, I have worked in the field of *Bioidentical Hormone Replacement Therapy (BHRT)*, seeing patients in medical clinics with physicians, speaking at medical conferences, and developing manuals and courses to train health care providers in BHRT. Essentially, all of my work has been in the secular marketplace where I have not had liberty to share my faith openly. You can't exactly pray out loud over your audience of three hundred medical doctors. Now, in this new season for me, I get the privilege of taking what He has taught me and the ministry He has birthed in me to His women. Words cannot even begin to describe the joy it brings to my heart.

Beyond professional experience, I have to admit that what really qualifies me to write a book about hormones is the fact that I can personally relate to what women go through. I know what it's like to have symptoms of hormone imbalance. Fifteen years ago, I was just a young woman with a serious case of premenstrual syndrome (PMS), which in Christian terms stands for **P**retty **M**ean **S**ister. I had mood swings and irritability before my period, premenstrual headaches that no medication seemed to help, acne, and many other

xvii

monthly symptoms. The misery drove me to find the cause and cor-responding solution, and once I found the help I needed, I couldn't help sharing it. I very soon realized that it was my passion to learn more and more about hormones. It's not my job; it is truly my God-given passion. I have given my life to it, and I'm delighted to go to the office each day to work with hormonally imbalanced women. That energy and dedication must be from God.

God Cares About Our Hormones

I am convinced that God is concerned about our hormone bal-ance or lack thereof. After all, He created these powerful chemicals in our bodies to play the amazing roles they were designed to play in perfect balance. God created menstrual cycles, not PMS. God ordained menopause, not hot flashes. I cannot prove it scientifically, but that certainly is my opinion. God never meant for His daugh-ters to suffer monthly or as the menstrual cycles stop. He is a good God. As you know, the devil perverts every good thing God does. God's plan is to launch women into kingdom ministries and for them to fulfill their callings as wives, mothers, and businesswomen. The impact He intends for women to have in the marketplace, in Christian circles, and in our personal lives is absolutely vital to the health of the body of Christ. He does not want anything like hor-mone problems to stand in our way. The enemy, on the other hand, would like nothing more than to take you out with hormone imbal-ances, to tempt you to scream at your kids or to have such bad night sweats that you can't sleep. If he can make you exhausted or give you hormonal headaches, he can slow you down and wreak havoc on your ministry in a variety of ways. Hormone imbalance is very real; so are its symptoms. Hot flashes aren't fatal, but certain family members could risk becoming fatalities if they say the wrong thing at the wrong time of the month. I don't think this suffering is God's best for us.

In the following chapters, I will cover the physical, mental, and emotional symptoms associated with hormone imbalances, but let me take time now to describe what I believe are some of the spiritual symptoms associated with hormone imbalance. Since hormones directly affect our emotions, hormone imbalances can cause symptoms such as inexplicable depression, irritability, anxiety, or mood swings—all of which can affect us spiritually. Women often experience guilt, shame, or condemnation over their feelings or behaviors during episodes of mood swings or irritability. It is hard for us to walk in love toward ourselves if hormonal imbalances are at the root of low self-esteem or lack of motivation. These feelings can trigger even more confusion, frustration, and isolation. I have heard many women with low hormone levels say that they just want to be left alone or that they just do not feel like being around people.

After all, we're supposed to walk in the fruit of the Spirit. Sometimes women just do not understand that hormone imbalances can make it very hard to do so. Countless women have told me they just do not feel like themselves when their hormones are out of balance, and believe me, I can surely relate. Certainly, we can't blame everything on hormones, but many times certain feelings *can* result from hormonal imbalance. If you find yourself dealing with issues that recur every month just before your menstrual period, consider the possibility of hormone-related problems. Sometimes the symptoms ease once the period starts, but sometimes they persist until about Day 7 of your cycle. If you begin noticing symptoms only as you approach your forties, or you suspect you are moving closer to menopause, or are even postmenopausal, these feelings could be hormone related. If you find yourself not acting like yourself, maybe your hormones—or lack thereof—are getting in your way.

Women this Book is Written for:

1. *Women who know they're struggling with hormone problems.*
2. *Women who wonder whether they have hormone problems.*
3. *Women of all ages who have hormone problems but don't know it.*
4. *Women taking traditional hormone replacement therapy (HRT), birth control pills or antidepressants/anti-anxiety medication to manage various hormone-related symptoms because they don't know there are better options.*

Do any of these descriptions fit your circumstance? Let me go into a bit of detail about each of these groups.

Group 1
Women who know they're struggling with hormone problems but don't know what to do about them.

I once had a patient whom I will call Rita. In the space on my intake form set aside for women to write what they would like to accomplish in working with me, she wrote words that really burden my heart still: "Since my surgery in November [she'd had a hysterectomy] with taking synthetic hormones, I have never felt right. My first month, December, was okay, but by mid-January, I felt stressed. By mid-February, I felt so anxious; I felt suicidal and described myself to my doctor: "I am PMS times three thousand. Despite exercise, my waist is thickening. I overreact to stress. I cry easily. I feel helpless and out of control. I just want to feel 'normal' again." As I have shared Rita's heartfelt plea at many women's conferences, numerous ladies have stood up and said that they could have written the very same words. Let me say again that I do not believe that God intends for us to have monthly misery or menopausal misery. Even women like Rita who have had hysterectomies are entitled to beautifully balanced hormones.

A lot of women are confused about hormones. As a speaker to women's groups and conferences for over a decade, I ask the same question everywhere I go: "Ladies, how many of you would say you are confused about hormones?" Inevitably hands go up all across the audience. Women in perimenopause or menopause ask questions as follows: Should I take hormones or not? Can the hormones cause cancer? If I don't take hormones, will I get osteoporosis? Is traditional HRT the only way to get rid of these miserable hot flashes? I'm afraid to stay on HRT, but then I'm afraid to stop taking it because the symptoms were so bad without it; what can I do? My doctor said the new low-dose HRT is safer; is it? Is it okay to take HRT for a couple of years just to get through menopause?

Most women in menopause who are scared of HRT are unaware that safer options exist, or they don't know how to avail themselves of these options. And the vast majority of women of all ages do not know the difference between synthetic hormones and natural, bioidentical hormones.

I have to say that while the news media usually does a great job of keeping us informed, in the case of hormones they have inadvertently contributed to the confusion. When reporting the results of hormone studies, they often don't specify the types of hormones the researchers studied. For example, when the widely reported Women's Health Initiative study in 2001 found that a popular HRT drug called Prempro® increased the risk of breast cancer, among other things, the news media made the incorrect blanket statement that estrogen and progesterone increase the risk of breast cancer. Make sure you understand this: *the Women's Health Initiative researchers **did not** study natural, human bioidentical estrogen and progesterone.* Prempro®, the drug they studied, is a combination of synthetic progesterone and conjugated equine estrogen, which is derived from pregnant mares' urine. Let me repeat: the researchers studied *horse* estrogen along with *synthetic* progesterone; these are very different from human and bioidentical hormones.

No wonder women are confused. Even many medical practitioners are confused about hormones. In my years of training medical doctors, nurse practitioners and physicians' assistants in BHRT, I have come to realize that many have not had the opportunity to learn the difference between bioidentical hormones and non-bioidentical hormones like Prempro® and Premarin®. Their confusion isn't surprising since too often even medical studies and literature written for health care professionals don't distinguish between bioidentical and non-bioidentical hormones. Sadly, because of this confusion, many women needlessly continue to tolerate some very unpleasant symptoms. Worse, some women suffer serious long-term consequences of hormone imbalances and deficiencies, including fibroid tumors, fibrocystic breast disease, osteoporosis, and breast cancer. (For a more complete list of symptoms and conditions related to hormone imbalances, please see Chapter 3.) The good news is that when they learn about the differences between traditional HRT and BHRT, many health-care providers are eager to learn how to prescribe BHRT for their patients.

Group 2
Women who wonder whether they have hormone problems.

Women in this group are pretty sure something is wrong, and they wonder whether their symptoms could be hormone related. A lot of them are hoping to find out they aren't crazy, and it is not all in their heads. They're frustrated because they're gaining weight while eating right or because they can't sleep any more. What could be causing their depression, waning sex drive, or migraines? Many women think that since they are not yet having hot flashes they can't be having hormone problems. Little do they know that most women experience a drop in progesterone during their thirties, causing a whole array of symptoms from headaches to breast cysts to weight gain. (See Chapter 3 for more symptoms of progesterone deficiency.) It is this lack of knowledge that keeps them from getting the progesterone supplementation they may need long before menopause.

Group 3
Women of all ages who have hormone problems but don't know it.

Again, most women think that as long as they aren't having hot flashes they can't be having hormone troubles. In addition to the symptoms mentioned above, many women suffer from hormonally induced menstrual distress, PMS, infertility, and miscarriages. Unfortunately, these correctable hormonal imbalances very often go undiagnosed and untreated, or they are treated with powerful synthetic hormones that can cause more problems than they fix. And then there are postmenopausal women who think they are "past all that." They've been told that osteoporosis, weight gain, insomnia, foggy thinking, and fatigue are all inevitable as they get older, and they'll just have to live with it. Not so. I have very good news for you, so keep reading. The information in this book can help you understand hormones and hormonal imbalance. You will also learn how to test accurately to detect hormonal imbalance.

Group 4
Women taking traditional hormone replacement therapy (HRT), birth control pills or antidepressants/anti-anxiety medication to manage various hormone-related symptoms because they don't know there are better options.

Many women, uncomfortable about taking Hormone Replacement Therapy (HRT), estrogen replacement therapy (ERT), and other medications have tried to tough it out without medication, but they just couldn't stand severe menopausal symptoms like incessant hot flashes. Not knowing about alternatives, they have reluctantly started taking HRT. And doctors often prescribe oral contraceptives to manage younger women's hormone-related symptoms and conditions. In some cases, doctors prescribe anti-depressant or anti-anxiety medications when women complain of PMS or menopause symptoms. Often, they do help. Sometimes they do not. The more important point, I think, is that these medications don't correct the underlying hormone imbalance. They are Band-Aids. Sometimes Band-Aids are good, but solving the underlying problem is better. I hope you are already beginning to see that there are safer and equally effective options to these traditional methods. Any woman currently taking HRT or oral contraceptives can easily switch to natural, bioidentical hormones.

Women Deserve Help

Watching women suffer and struggle needlessly because they don't know about safe, viable solutions drives me to get the word out. The symptoms of hormonal imbalance are very real. I say that it does not have to be like this. Having experienced the symptoms firsthand, I will not sit quietly by and watch women go without information and help. It is like a fire shut in my bones, and the only way to quench it is to keep speaking, writing, teaching, and finding other ways to preach this gospel of help and hope for women. Learning the truth is the way for women to be set free. Proclaiming this truth is and will remain my destiny for the rest of my days. If "…all things work together for good to them that love God, to them who are called according to his purpose," then personally enduring such severe hormone imbalance was worthwhile because now I get to see the lives of other women transformed and restored to the fullness that Jesus purchased for us with His very life (Rom. 8:28).

It is just like God to work all things together for our good and to allow us to comfort others with the same comfort we have been comforted with. He turned my mess into my ministry. I clearly see that it was God who took my career and put me in places and positions that I could never have attained on my own. I also know that He did it so that I could help Him take care of His daughters.

Overcoming Hormone Imbalance Is Possible

We can have victory over hormone imbalance. If we perish for lack of knowledge, what sets us free? The world says information is power; I say that all we need is TRUTH and the Holy Spirit will lead and guide us into all truth. I have made every attempt to share truth, science and my clinical experience in order to give you the keys that will make sure you overcome symptoms of hormone imbalance and improve the quality of your life. This sums up quite well my intention in writing to you. The motive of my heart in my life's work is to provide truth that will help women struggling with symptoms and diseases associated with hormone problems.

My mission statement: to educate, encourage, and equip women in the area of hormone balance. I hope this book does just that for you.

Chapter 1

DO YOU NEED A HORMONE MAKEOVER?

Since hormones affect every cell in your body, it's hardly surprising that hormone excesses, deficiencies, or imbalances can produce some very unpleasant, debilitating, and even dangerous symptoms. For example, hormones affect your cardiovascular system, central nervous system, blood sugar balance, bone density, weight, and skin, to list a few.

Hormones also affect brain function and mood. Therefore, hormone imbalances, especially sex hormone imbalances, can impair mental sharpness, ability to focus, and short-term memory, making you feel like your brain is in a fog. At the same time, mood swings, irritability, depression, and anxiety may increase—a dreadful combination. Needless to say, this sort of thing can be pretty rough on your career, relationships, and all other areas of your life.

Here are a few questions to help you decide whether you might need a hormone makeover. If you answer yes to any of these questions, go through the checklist for a more comprehensive assessment.

Questions to Consider:

➢ Have you gained weight, especially around the abdomen or hips?
➢ Are you having hot flashes or night sweats?

> ➤ Have your menstrual cycles become irregular, become too heavy, or recently stopped? What about hormonal headaches or migraines?
> ➤ How about your skin—has it become very dry or too oily?
> ➤ Has your doctor told you that you have lost bone mass?
> ➤ Are you having trouble remembering what you went to the pantry for or even your best friend's name?
> ➤ Do you have "brain fog"?
> ➤ Have you lost interest in physical intimacy, or are you having trouble sleeping?
> ➤ In addition to these physical and mental symptoms, have you experienced unexplained depression or weepiness?
> ➤ Have you felt more anxious, stressed, or irritable?
> ➤ Have you had a hysterectomy and found that you have not been the same since?

If you answered yes to any of these questions, let me give you some good news: you don't have to live with these symptoms. Maybe you just need a hormone makeover. And if so, you are not alone. In fact, right now about forty million women in the United States are in menopause, and 80 to 90% of women of childbearing age report PMS symptoms.

As women enter their thirties, hormone levels typically begin to fall, often triggering menstrual symptoms as well as afflictions like weight gain, headaches, lack of sex drive, and depression, just to name a few. Unfortunately, it doesn't get any better as women move into their forties and fifties. Instead, they tend to get even *more* annoying symptoms like hot flashes, night sweats, vaginal dryness, brain fog, and insomnia. Left unattended, some types of hormone imbalances can even result in bone loss, breast cysts, uterine fibroids, and a higher risk of cardiovascular disease. Clearly, hormone imbalances aren't problems you should just suffer through or try to ignore.

Hormone Imbalance Checklist

As you complete the following checklist, please keep in mind that the symptoms in each category do overlap. It can be confusing, but a BHRT specialist can help you sort through your symptoms and test your saliva to measure your estrogen, progesterone, testosterone, Dehydroepiandrosterone (DHEA), and cortisol levels. He or she will also test your blood to determine thyroid hormone and blood sugar levels.

Symptoms of Hormone Deficiencies

1. Symptoms of Progesterone Deficiency

Progesterone deficiency often occurs by the mid-thirties, often dropping by about 75% between the mid-thirties and menopause. Since progesterone is produced by the ovaries, women whose ovaries have been removed are likely to be progesterone deficient. Also, women on birth control pills, patches, or injections are not allowed to ovulate. That is how these birth control methods work. However, ovulation must take place in order for women to produce appreciable amounts of progesterone.

General Physical Symptoms or Related Conditions:
- ☐ Weight gain
- ☐ Fluid retention
- ☐ Low body temperature
- ☐ Hypothyroidism (under-activity of the thyroid gland)
- ☐ Headaches
- ☐ Pain and inflammation
- ☐ Allergies/sinusitis
- ☐ Insomnia or sleep disturbances
- ☐ Hair loss
- ☐ Bone loss

Gynecological Symptoms or Related Conditions:
- ☐ PMS

- ☐ Cramps
- ☐ Breast pain/benign cysts
- ☐ Heavy periods
- ☐ Irregular cycles (periods too close together)
- ☐ Spotting before period or break-through bleeding
- ☐ Fibroids
- ☐ Endometriosis
- ☐ Infertility
- ☐ Miscarriage
- ☐ Luteal phase deficiency (a common cause of infertility)

Emotional Symptoms or Related Conditions:
- ☐ Depression
- ☐ Anxiety
- ☐ Irritability
- ☐ Mood swings
- ☐ Tendency to be stressed easily

2. Symptoms of Estrogen Deficiency

Estrogen deficiency or estrogen deficiency symptoms due to lower levels may occur during mid to late forties or early fifties and are more likely to occur under conditions of long term chronic stress. Women whose ovaries have been removed are also likely to be estrogen deficient unless they are on some type of estrogen replacement therapy.

General Physical Symptoms or Related Conditions:
- ☐ Vasomotor symptoms: hot flashes/night sweats
- ☐ Headaches
- ☐ Insomnia or sleep disturbances
- ☐ Poor memory/concentration or forgetfulness
- ☐ Hair loss
- ☐ Dry skin/eyes/hair
- ☐ Thinning/aging skin and wrinkles
- ☐ Bone loss
- ☐ Insulin resistance
- ☐ Oily skin/acne

☐ Weight gain
☐ Heart palpitations

Gynecological Symptoms or Related Conditions:
☐ Lighter/non-existent periods
☐ Vaginal dryness
☐ Painful intercourse
☐ Urinary tract infections
☐ Incontinence

Emotional Symptoms or Related Conditions:
☐ Depression
☐ Weepiness
☐ Anxiety
☐ Carbohydrate cravings
☐ Sleep disturbances
☐ Low libido

3. Symptoms of Testosterone Deficiency

Testosterone deficiency is very common in women whose ovaries have been removed. It may also occur as women approach menopause or are under situations of long-term chronic stress.

General Physical Symptoms or Related Conditions:
☐ Vasomotor symptoms: hot flashes/night sweats
☐ Aches and pains
☐ Fatigue
☐ Insomnia
☐ Poor memory
☐ Thinning skin
☐ Loss of muscle tone
☐ Bone loss
☐ Heart palpitations

Gynecological Symptoms or Related Conditions:
☐ Loss or thinning of pubic hair
☐ Vaginal dryness
☐ Incontinence

☐ Lichen sclerosis
☐ Loss of libido
☐ Impaired sexual function or female sexual arousal disorder

Emotional Symptoms or Related Conditions:
☐ Depression
☐ Lack of motivation

4. Symptoms of Thyroid Hormone Deficiency

Thyroid hormone deficiency is called hypothyroidism. For an extensive explanation, see Chapter 5.

☐ Weight gain
☐ Difficulty losing weight
☐ Exhaustion
☐ Lack of energy
☐ Excessive sleeping
☐ Sleep disturbances
☐ Low body temperature
☐ Intolerance of cold
☐ Cold hands and feet
☐ Decreased sweating
☐ Depression, mild to severe
☐ Memory loss
☐ Fuzzy thinking
☐ Difficulty following conversations or losing train of thought
☐ Slowness or slurring of speech
☐ Slowed reflexes
☐ Brittle nails
☐ Brittle hair
☐ Hair loss
☐ Thinning or loss of sides of eyebrows
☐ Itchy scalp
☐ Dry skin
☐ Thinning skin
☐ Persistent cold sores, boils, or pimples
☐ Orange-colored soles and palms

☐ Joint and muscle pain
☐ Carpal tunnel syndrome
☐ Tingling sensation in wrists and hands that mimics carpal tunnel syndrome
☐ Low blood pressure
☐ Slow pulse
☐ Heart palpitations
☐ Blood clotting problems
☐ Bruising
☐ Elevated LDL (the "bad" cholesterol)
☐ Irregular periods
☐ PMS
☐ Diminished sex drive
☐ Infertility
☐ Miscarriage
☐ Breast milk formation
☐ Headaches
☐ Allergies (sudden appearance or worsening)
☐ Hoarseness
☐ Puffiness in face and extremities
☐ Constipation
☐ Calcium metabolism difficulties resulting in leg cramps or bone loss

5. Symptoms of Cortisol Deficiency

Cortisol is made by the adrenal glands. If the body has been under long-term chronic stress, cortisol production may be compromised.

☐ Fatigue or chronic fatigue syndrome
☐ Stress
☐ Irritability
☐ Low blood sugar or hypoglycemia (feelings of shakiness, weakness, headache, or irritability if you miss a meal)
☐ Low body temperature
☐ Sugar cravings
☐ Chemical sensitivity

☐ Heart palpitations
☐ Aches/pains such as muscle or joint pain
☐ Arthritis
☐ Allergies

Symptoms of Hormone Excesses

1. Symptoms of Excess Estrogen

Estrogen and progesterone complement each other; that is, each hormone counteracts the effects of the other to create a harmonious balance. The collection of symptoms related to excess estrogen relative to progesterone is called estrogen dominance. Please see Chapter 3 for a discussion of estrogen dominance. This imbalance occurs when there's not enough progesterone to balance estrogen. A woman may not necessarily have excess levels of estrogen to be estrogen dominant; she may simply have relatively high estrogen levels compared with her progesterone level. Before treatment, the symptoms listed below can be confirmed by lab tests showing a low progesterone-to-estradiol ratio.

☐ Weight gain
☐ Fluid retention
☐ Symptoms of hypothyroidism
☐ Hormonal and premenstrual headaches
☐ Other headaches
☐ Irritability
☐ Sleep disturbances
☐ Low libido
☐ Breast pain, fibrocystic breast disease, breast cancer, breast adenomas
☐ Irregular bleeding
☐ Heavy bleeding
☐ Blood clots in menstrual flow
☐ Uterine fibroids
☐ Endometriosis

2. Symptoms of Excess Progesterone

Excess progesterone is always a result of taking too much supplemental progesterone; the body itself never over-produces progesterone.

- ☐ Sleepiness
- ☐ Bloating
- ☐ Candida
- ☐ Estrogen deficiency symptoms

3. Symptoms of Excess Testosterone

- ☐ Acne/oily skin
- ☐ Facial hair
- ☐ Thinning scalp hair
- ☐ Excess body hair
- ☐ Mid-cycle pain (at ovulation)
- ☐ Pain in nipples
- ☐ Ovarian cysts
- ☐ Hypoglycemia or insulin resistance
- ☐ Elevated triglycerides
- ☐ Aggression, irritability

4. Symptoms of Excess Cortisol

Chronic excessive stress can lead to chronic over-production of cortisol.

- ☐ Insomnia/sleep disturbances
- ☐ Headaches
- ☐ "Tired but wired" feeling
- ☐ Stressed feeling
- ☐ Irritability
- ☐ Low libido
- ☐ Depression
- ☐ Food cravings

☐ Low serotonin (causes depression and carbohydrate cravings)

☐ Hormone resistance (meaning that the body is unable to properly use any or all of these hormones: thyroid, insulin, estrogen, testosterone and progesterone, causing symptoms of deficiencies of these hormones)

☐ Thinning skin

☐ Loss of muscle mass

☐ Bone loss

☐ Heart palpitations

☐ Cardiovascular disease

☐ Breast cancer

Please bear in mind that diagnosis or therapy should not rely on symptoms alone. Proper hormone testing is *essential* to determining and then correcting the underlying hormone imbalances causing the symptoms. And don't be discouraged if you found yourself checking a lot of boxes on the checklist. Isn't it a relief to discover that so many odd, seemingly unrelated physical and emotional symptoms may actually stem from the same underlying problem? This is especially true since hormone imbalances are usually easy to correct. The truth sets us free, or as some would say, "Knowledge is power." So be encouraged; help is available as you can see from the following real life hormone makeovers. These ladies recognized they needed help and reached out to get it. Read on to be inspired.

Real Women That Needed and Got "The Hormone Makeover"

What better way to help explain the impact of hormonal imbalance than to have real women share their hormone makeover stories? The following ladies willingly wrote their own accounts because they wanted other women to know what difference bioidentical hormones can make. Each precious story is literally in the woman's own words and has not been edited or changed. You are going to enjoy each one. After each lady's note, I will share commentary on the types of hormones each one takes. Perhaps this will help further explain their responses.

A.B.'s Hormone Makeover
Age 47

For years I had long, heavy, frequent periods, so I eventually became seriously anemic and depressed. Not realizing I was anemic, I thought I was lazy and hated myself for it. I also had really bad PMS—I was irritable and horribly depressed. Later I began to experience symptoms of estrogen deficiency: hot flashes that lasted for hours at a time, memory problems, and terrible brain fog that almost cost me my job.

Based on my saliva test results, Donna and her physician got me started on bioidentical estrogen and progesterone, and all my symptoms resolved very quickly. Sleeping through the night without waking up soaked in sweat was a lovely relief, and I looked more professional at work with my hair and clothes no longer drenched. My memory improved and the fog lifted so that I became very competent at work. My boss sure noticed a huge improvement.

A few years later, as a result of stress at work and in my personal life, my cortisol level skyrocketed to three times the normal level, and I sure had the symptoms. I couldn't sleep; I was easily startled, and I felt very much on edge. I just generally felt awful and couldn't think. Donna recommended some nutritional supplements that caused my cortisol levels to drop back to normal, and since then, I sleep great and am not at all easily upset. My brain works much better too. My hormone makeover revolutionized my life.

A.B.'s hormones: 0.025 mg estradiol patch, 20 mg of progesterone cream once daily, basic supplementation, and phosphatidylserine to manage her elevated cortisol.

A.G.'s Hormone Makeover
Age 39

I have personally used Donna White's "Hormone Makeover" services and also as a referral for my patients as a health professional.

In both areas, her services have shined. For me personally, I cannot say enough. I am in my late thirties, and Donna and her physician worked with me years ago on my hormones, which were literally all over the place. She got me on a wonderful regimen of progesterone and natural supplements. It made a world of difference. Not only did I feel more leveled out with my moods and energy, but I also started to ovulate on a very regular basis. This regularity was the best blessing of all because soon (after years of doctors telling me I may not be able to conceive) I was able to conceive NATURALLY. I stayed on the progesterone during and after pregnancy and swear that it helped me with adjusting as a new mom. While I hear moms experience some post partum depression, I experience nothing but feelings of joy. I can't help but contribute this to my hormones being leveled out.

As a health professional, I have referred to Donna many of my patients who were at a stand-still with their weight. They were very frustrated and were doing all of the right steps nutritionally, but my gut told me it was their hormones—out of experience and some of the charts and guidelines Donna had taught me. Sure enough, after meeting with Donna and doing the saliva test, clients were coming back to me with grins on their faces, more energy, better control over food cravings, less depression, and less irritability. It was and still is amazing. I love how they are getting the help they need via natural supplements and hormones.

I personally am honored to know and be able to work with Donna on both levels (personal and business). Her expertise and genuine care for others shines right through her, and you just know sitting with her that she truly does care and will do all she can to get to the bottom of the problem. I am blessed to have her in my life.

A.G.'s hormones: 30 mg of Armour Thyroid daily and 20 mg of progesterone cream daily on Days 7-28 of her cycle.

K.P.'s Hormone Makeover
Age 48

I just want to thank you for all your help and advice that has truly changed my life. Before I came to see you and your doctor,

I was suffering from terrible dizzy spells, heart palpitations during the day and night, hot flashes, and trouble sleeping. I was extremely tired and had no energy. After wearing a heart monitor, having several EKG's, an ultrasound of my heart, stress tests, and blood tests, I was diagnosed with depression and given an anti-depressant.

Well, that was not good enough for me since I was not depressed and refused to take anti-depressants. I saw a sign for one of your Hormone Makeover Seminars and after attending and immediately making an appointment to see you, my life changed for the better.

You immediately suggested a saliva test which is much more reliable and informative for hormone levels than a blood test. My results showed that my thyroid was unproductive. I had very low progesterone levels, high testosterone levels, and I did not need the estrogen my male gynecologist had prescribed; my body made plenty on its own. (Estrogen supplementation seems to be the number one cure doctors like to prescribe for all women with hormone problems, whether they need it or not.) I also needed to increase my vitamin C, calcium, and iron; easy vitamins to take; no prescriptions needed.

With these simple, healthy changes, I feel so much better and have lots of energy. I did not need to take any anti-depressants.

Every chance I get, I recommend you to all my friends who have many similar problems that I had, with no results from all the tests their current doctors run them through. Thank you again, Donna, for all of your help.

K.P.'s hormones: Thyrolar 2, 30 mg of progesterone cream daily, 5 mg capsules of DHEA once daily, along with supplements to help with insulin resistance and reduce testosterone (N-A-C).

M.M.'s Hormone Makeover
Age 59

For several years prior to using bioidentical hormones, I took hormone replacement therapy prescribed by my physician. When the government study was published, which indicated that women who used synthetic hormones were more susceptible to heart attacks and strokes, I discontinued the treatment.

I took herbs, which helped somewhat, but I still had some problems with hot flashes, low energy, and low libido. Since taking bioidentical hormones prescribed by Donna White's medical providers, I feel much better. My energy level has increased significantly as well as my libido, and I do not experience hot flashes.

M.M.'s hormones: Biest Cream at 0.1mg (70% Estriol, 30% Estradiol) compounded with 30 mg of progesterone and 0.1 mg of testosterone along with 90 mg of Armour thyroid.

D.P.'s Hormone Makeover
Age 45

My name is "Diane," and I am forty-five years old. The hormone-related symptoms I experienced began in my late thirties but increasingly became worse by the time I was forty-three. One night while I was lying on the couch with my hands resting near my throat, I discovered a lump on the front of my neck. I made an appointment to see my family doctor the next day. He ran thyroid tests and an ultrasound to measure the lump—later diagnosed as a goiter. The thyroid test results came back within a range where it was explained that no treatment was necessary, and I was told there was nothing I could do about the goiter (that the lump was not likely to go away). My original symptoms further worsened and now included a racing heart, sleeplessness, anxiety, depression, muscle aches, headaches, and more difficult periods with blood clots. I confided in several of my menopause-aged friends to ask them questions about their experiences. They were very supportive and said much of what I described sounded similar to what they were going through or had already experienced.

Convinced I was entering menopause, I began to read books, educate myself, research, and watch television programs featuring information about its symptoms. I wanted to prepare myself, or should I say "brace" myself, for the inevitable.

I was always a healthy person, but the symptoms I was having made me feel like I was losing my mind. I did not have PMS like many of my friends. I did not have mood swings or other symptoms. At this time, however, I had to begin "talking myself off the ledge" every month at the end of my period when heightened anxiety and depression set in. I was getting little sleep and my mind would not shut down when I tried to rest. I put a pen and paper by my bedside so I could write down the thoughts whizzing through my mind in the middle of the night. There were times when tears would flow for what seemed like no logical reason. Many days I would think, "What is the matter with me? There isn't anything going on in my life situationally that would explain the emotions I am having."

I consulted with my family doctor again and explained that I thought I was going through perimenopause and experiencing what appeared to be hormonal symptoms I could track each month with my cycle. I asked if there was any kind of test I could get to show what my hormones were doing. I was told there was not a test available. He listened to me describe my symptoms, but then suggested three prescriptions to solve my problems: 1) Zoloft for anxiety and depression 2) Birth Control Pills for difficult periods and 3) Ambien to help me sleep. It was suggested that I write down when I could expect to feel the worst symptoms on the calendar and mentally "deal with it" as part of my changing body. He was unable to piece together the other clues and information in my medical chart. I tried Ambien and several other types of sleep aids, and none helped me get a good night sleep. The entire experience did not feel right to me. I sensed something was wrong with the treatments offered to me, but I needed help to find out the root causes. I felt like my doctor was trying to put a Band-Aid on the problems, and I left feeling very discouraged.

A month or so after seeing the doctor, I was at a brunch with a good friend who asked me how I was doing. I explained what happened at the doctor, and she suggested I set up a consultation with Donna, a hormone education specialist. I learned she had a saliva test that determined hormone levels, which sounded worth trying. I was apprehensive of the cost, but I felt so bad most of the time that I was willing to take a chance. I prefer alternative medicines and approaches when it makes sense, but it is also difficult because treatment is not covered by insurance. As women, sometimes we put ourselves and our needs last which is a big mistake. If we are healthy, we will have more to give to the other relationships and activities in our lives.

I called the office to make an appointment and meticulously filled out the paperwork for the consultation. As I read the questions, I began to feel hope, even based on the information being requested, that Donna might have answers that my doctor did not. I was right in what I thought because it is exactly what resulted from my first consultation. Donna explained what I had been experiencing was *not* normal and was *not* something I should have to suffer with on an ongoing basis. I felt relieved. Donna took the time to listen to all of the different symptoms I was having and pieced them together like a puzzle. In my particular case, the hormonal-based symptoms I described pointed to a thyroid issue, not menopause. She also suspected, very common for my age, that I might have a progesterone deficiency.

After my consultation was over, we worked with the medical doctor on staff to "apply the science" to Donna's hypothesis. I was actually diagnosed with a thyroid disorder called Hashimoto's Disease. It is possible my thyroid had not worked properly for many years, and I would have continued to live with horrible symptoms the rest of my life if it were not for the help I received. The separate saliva test also showed high levels of estrogen resulting in a progesterone deficiency. Within the first week of taking the thyroid replacement hormones, I no longer experienced anxiety or depression. Almost 50% of my symptoms were gone within a couple more weeks. My entire life felt back on track, and I felt like myself again for the first time in years.

We are still in the process of determining the correct doses to treat my issues, and it requires patience to work through the details of Hashimoto's Disease. I am glad I did not give up and that I followed my instincts to pursue the root causes for the symptoms I was experiencing. Because of this positive experience, I no longer fear menopause. I know there is a way to measure hormone levels and that compounding pharmacies are available to provide bioidentical hormone replacement in lieu of synthetic drugs. Thank you, Donna, for your expertise and patience in helping us find the right treatment(s) to bring us optimal health.

D.P.'s hormones: Synthroid 25 mcg and 5 mcg of Cytomel thyroid medications, 20 mg of progesterone cream, and Indole-3-Carbinol supplement to reduce and metabolize elevated estrogen.

J.G.'s Hormone Makeover
Age 45

Thirteen years ago, I had a total hysterectomy, and when I was going through it all, my gynecologist did not even mention that it would put me into immediate surgical menopause. But within a week after surgery, I started with the hot flashes and crying almost all the time. He then did put me on an oral estrogen. As a couple years went by, I kept inquiring as to why estrogen only and no other hormones. And their reply was always the same thing: you don't need progesterone if you no longer have a uterus. So I went for a decade with what I can presume to be estrogen dominance. Therefore, I developed many of those symptoms such as weight gain, mood swings, sugar cravings, and severe breast pain. About five years ago, I started trying to get my specialist to test my hormones, and he would only run blood tests, which came back in what they called a normal range. I tried to get them to run saliva tests, and I was just laughed at. So I was left on estrogen alone.

Finally at a primary care specialist, I was introduced to Donna White, a BHRT Clinical Education Consultant. Donna provided education on how to properly test and treat hormones and their related imbalances. I learned that saliva testing allowed us to see what hormones were actually getting out to my tissues, etc. And also on saliva testing, we could test while I was on different hormones to see how they affected my ranges. My testing showed marked hormonal imbalance. So I was immediately switched to bioidentical hormones. Compounded progesterone was added, and my estrogen was changed to a patch. Within the first week, I became noticeably less depressed, and I had a marked decrease in anxiety and tremendous improvement in food cravings. And once I started on the progesterone, I noticed that I could concentrate and think more clearly. And over the next year, I lost eighteen pounds without even changing my diet. People are always asking me what I have done to my face, too, because they say my skin looks so much better, and I look younger. Also, for years doctors have been trying to get my adrenal health to improve to no avail. It took a couple of years on the BHRT, but now my adrenals have come back to life on their own. Before BHRT, I was on antidepressants, sleep, pain, and anxiety medication. Now I don't have to take any of those. My life has totally changed thanks to BHRT.

I would like to encourage women to help themselves with this type of testing and treatment. Remember the old saying, "If mamma ain't happy, ain't no one happy"? If we don't take care of ourselves, it will inhibit our ability to take care of our family and enjoy life. But I would also like to point out that women should remember their daughters and realize this can benefit them too. When I was in high school, I had such horrible menstrual periods that my mom had to take me out of school and work for several days a month. I would lie in bed, literally screaming from the pain. And I wasn't all that polite during the weeks before my cycle. If my mom had known about BHRT, she could have helped me find out that perhaps my estrogen and progesterone needed tweaking during the month, and I could have had a much happier, healthier adolescence, which we all know is a hard enough time without female problems.

J.G.'s hormones: 0.1mg estradiol patch 2 x weekly, 40 mg progesterone cream once daily, and one compounded sustained-release thyroid T3 capsule daily.

A.L.'s Hormone Makeover
Age 45

In my early forties, I had been having trouble sleeping and had horrible migraines lasting three to four days, two to three times monthly. After three years of working towards a master's degree, I attributed much of this pain to stress and the late nights of studying. I was also struggling with some symptoms of depression, which I thought was the result of a recent move across half the country. In addition, I had absolutely NO sex-drive. Then, I began waking up in the middle of the night, soaking wet with sweat and needing to peel off my clothes to get comfortable. And, if this weren't enough to deal with, I began putting on weight around my mid-section.

I read several books by Suzanne Sommers and Louise Gittleman on peri-menopause. I began to research Bioidentical Hormone Replacement Therapy (BHRT). I started with a doctor who advertised this specialty. He tested hormone levels through blood tests and determined that I was low in testosterone and progesterone. I began oral BHRT. After almost two years of this, I was still not feeling like I thought I should. I still had no energy, a low sex-drive, and I felt angry all the time.

I decided to pursue another professional who could re-evaluate my hormone needs. Donna had me do the saliva test, and she explained why it was a better method of testing. In addition, she explained why topical progesterone would be better utilized into my body rather than the oral. When the test results came back, my estrogen was very high, my progesterone was still relatively low, and my testosterone was off the charts high. I had been taking almost as much testosterone as a grown man makes in his body. Donna was able to help my doctor bring my estrogen and testosterone back into normal levels. And, the change to topical progesterone helped me as well. Today, I am pretty much symptom free.

Through this I have learned that I know my body pretty well, and I know when things are "out of whack." I have learned that when I am not getting satisfactory answers, I need to keep researching and talking to professionals until I get what I need. I am thankful for the people, like Donna, that God has placed in my path and that have helped me so much.

A.L.'s hormones: 20 mg of Progesterone cream on Days 7-28 of her cycle, soy isoflavones 60 mg daily and DHEA 10 mg orally.

E.S.'s Hormone Makeover
Age 46

I am a forty-six year old woman who has suffered from hormonal imbalances since my early twenties; however, when I was younger, my symptoms were much milder. About a week before my period, I would feel bloated, sluggish, and crave chocolate. (I would make a batch of brownies and eat the whole thing.) A few days before my period, I might feel a little sad and melancholy for no reason. I would also experience mild to moderate cramps for a few days.

However after the birth of each of my three children, my symptoms worsened. About a week before my period, I was bloated, exhausted, had extreme anxiety, mild depression, and trouble sleeping. The brain fog that I would occasionally experience was extremely unsettling. I remember driving in my car and forgetting where I was going. I just wasn't thinking clearly. The day before my period, I cried on and off for no particular reason. My physical symptoms were also debilitating. I couldn't leave the house for the first two days; the blood flow was so heavy that I had to construct makeshift diapers.

In 1992, I had some ovarian cysts that ruptured and my doctor put me on five days of progesterone, followed by three months of the birth control pill. I felt horrible on these hormones; I was constantly nauseated, and I gained ten pounds. I knew that I would never go on synthetic hormones. In 2001, I had an endometrial ablation to alleviate the heavy bleeding I experienced each month. It worked in the sense that I no longer bled each month, but I still had all of my other symptoms.

Throughout the years, I had tried various supplements and healthy ways of eating with little success. I still had two bad weeks a month—the week before my period and the week of. As the years unfolded, my symptoms became more unbearable, with extreme fatigue, depression, and occasional hot flashes and night sweats. I felt like I had one foot in the grave.

I first found out about Donna at my doctor's office. I saw her pamphlet, and I felt hope for the first time in a long time. I bought the test kit and waited for my results. I was so impressed with Donna. Here was a woman who actually listened to me and asked many questions. She looked at the whole picture and really dug deep to find out what was going on. My estrogen and progesterone levels were very low, and my testosterone level was very high. My adrenals were also shot. Donna also suggested that the doctor test my thyroid. Donna's doctors prescribed progesterone cream, N-Acetyl Cysteine (to lower the testosterone), various supplements, and dietary changes.

I was also diagnosed with hypothyroidism and went on a low dose of Armour thyroid. Within a few months, I was feeling much better and saw occasional glimpses of my old self. Months later, I retested and returned to see Donna. Her doctor added a low-dose estrogen patch. I really feel like that was the missing piece of the puzzle. I have been on the estrogen patch for almost three months, and I feel better than I have in years. I went to pick up my estrogen prescription the other day, and I told my pharmacist, "I feel so much better; there are days where I feel like I am in my twenties." I think much more clearly. I am much calmer and enjoy life again. I am so grateful! Thank you, Donna!

E.S.'s hormones: 20 mg of progesterone cream on Days 7-28 of her cycle, 0.025 mg estradiol patch, and 25 mcg of Synthroid.

T.B.'s Hormone Makeover
Age 55

I'd always joked that hot flashes would be a welcomed relief from the cold hands and feet I normally struggled with. Little did I know how miserable they really are. The biggest problem was getting enough sleep due to night sweats. During the day, without warning, I'd be drenched by what I came to call "spontaneous combustion." Quality of life takes a huge nosedive when hormones go away.

But the hot flashes proved to be less disturbing than the weight gain from an underactive thyroid. No matter how hard I worked out, I couldn't make a difference. And I was blown away by the fact that western medicine interprets thyroid numbers totally different from the naturopathic point of view. Once that was under control, I began to feel like my old self again.

T.B.'s hormones: 0.05 mg estradiol patch, 10 mg of progesterone cream compounded with 1 mg of DHEA, and Thyrolar 2.

You can have a fantastic hormone makeover story too.
Keep reading.

Chapter 2

YOUR FOUR OPTIONS

If you're experiencing symptoms of hormonal imbalances or deficiencies or if you're concerned about their long-term health effects, it seems to me that you have four options: use bioidentical hormone replacement therapy (BHRT), take traditional hormone replacement therapy (HRT or ERT, which is estrogen only therapy), use over-the-counter (OTC) remedies, or just try to cope with symptoms. Let's look at each of these possible choices.

More About*:*

Definitions: Therapy Options to Manage Hormone Imbalance

BHRT - *The use of biologically identical hormones, also called human-identical, because the molecular shape is an exact match to the hormones the body produces. They act and perform exactly like the human hormones because they, indeed, are exactly the same.*

HRT - *Typically the use of hormones to address symptoms of hormone deficiency usually consisting of some form of* *estrogen-either synthetic, animal derived, or biologically identical-along with synthetic progesterone.*

ERT *- The use of some form of estrogen (synthetic, animal derived or biologically identical) without progesterone. It is usually prescribed for women who have had their ovaries removed.*

OTC *- Over-the-counter supplements containing various ingredients, usually phytoestrogens (plant derived chemicals similar to estrogens), which may offset symptoms of hormone imbalance.*

Option 1

BHRT: Bioidentical Hormone Replacement Therapy

BHRT refers to the supplementation of endogenous (produced by the body) estrogen and progesterone with bioidentical hormones to correct imbalances and deficiencies, just as doctors prescribe thyroid or insulin to make up a shortfall in the body's production. Derived from soy and yams through a process discovered in 1942 by an American chemist, bioidentical hormones have been used safely and successfully in Europe for over sixty years. BHRT is not hormone mega-dosing, but it is the restoration of normal levels of hormones a healthy woman should produce. It is not a one-dose-fits-all approach. BHRT practitioners test hormone levels before and after starting therapy to ensure proper dosing, knowing that individual physiological differences and differences in life situations affect needs. Some women's bodies are very sensitive and need only minimal amounts of supplemental hormones, while others need a great deal more to achieve noticeable improvement. Stress levels and diet can also affect a woman's hormone needs, so BHRT professionals carefully tailor treatment to each woman.

Many people use the terms natural and bioidentical interchangeably, but the term bioidentical is more accurate because though bioidentical hormones are exactly like endogenous hormones, not all natural hormones are bioidentical. For example, equine (horse) estrogen is natural, but it isn't identical to human estrogen. Phytoestrogens are also natural but not identical to endogenous human estrogen.

The great thing about bioidentical hormones is that since their molecular structures perfectly match those of endogenous hormones, they function exactly like endogenous hormones do. Simply stated, bioidentical hormones do precisely the same thing as our own hormones.

More About:

The Hormone Cascade

This diagram shows the flow of hormones as they descend through the hormone cascade. All of the steroid hormones are synthesized from cholesterol into the hormones below. On the left hand side is progesterone, which can be converted into the hormones that fall beneath it, as shown by the arrows. On the right you see the hormones that are synthesized from DHEA. This diagram demonstrates that hormones can be converted into others. An excess or deficient level of any one of these hormones can affect the others.

Hormone Cascade

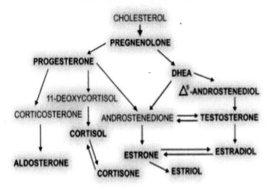

Advantages of BHRT

My philosophy on BHRT is to follow human physiology as closely as possible. In other words, put back what should be there in the proper amount based on age. Because bioidentical hormones function exactly like our own hormones, they follow an identical metabolic cascade, forming the same essential metabolites (the by-products of metabolism). Bioidentical hormones require the same enzymes for this metabolic process as endogenous hormones do. Again the point is that bioidentical hormones function exactly the same as human hormones.

Because bioidentical hormones are indistinguishable from endogenous hormones, BHRT, unlike traditional HRT, actually corrects hormone deficiencies and resolves the symptoms of the deficiency. As I said before, there's none of the one-dose-fits-all approach in BHRT; instead, BHRT is tailored to fit each woman's needs. And your BHRT practitioner will prescribe only those hormones you actually need and only in the amounts needed to restore balance and prevent disease. Testing ensures dosing accuracy and makes monitoring hormone levels easy. BHRT professionals should also address related health issues such as diet, stress hormones, and appropriate supplementation. Add to all this good news the fact that clinical reports by providers using BHRT indicate that BHRT causes virtually *no* side effects when used *properly* and the fact that we have a long history of safe use of BHRT. Speaking of safety, women have had estrogen, progesterone, and testosterone in their bodies since Eve was on earth. Think about it, these same hormones are at very high levels during puberty. (Do you remember how great that felt?) Not coincidentally, even with the higher levels during puberty, teenage girls are not at high risk of breast cancer.

More About:

Commonly Used Bioidentical Hormones:

Estrogens: estradiol and estriol
Progesterone
Testosterone
DHEA
Cortisol (hydrocortisone)
Pregnenolone
Melatonin
Thyroid
Insulin
Vitamin D (it is actually a hormone)

This is all great news, but what can BHRT actually *do* for you? BHRT is believed to or has been shown to:

- Reduce hot flashes, night sweats, and vaginal dryness
- Help maintain muscle mass and strength
- Help restore bone strength and prevent osteoporosis
- Alleviate depression and anxiety
- Improve mood, concentration, and memory
- Enhance sleep

- Increase libido
- Reduce the risk of breast and endometrial cancer*
- Protect against heart disease and stroke*
- Improve cholesterol levels
- Protect against senility and Alzheimer's disease*
- Produce far fewer side effects than traditional HRT when used properly

These have not been demonstrated with HRT.

Is it any wonder that an estimated 90-96% of women who begin BHRT stick with it? Not only that, women on hormones actually live longer, according to research. Okay, but here is the real question, "Is BHRT safe?" Opponents of BHRT frequently mention that there is no research indicating that BHRT is any safer than HRT. By the way, HRT has proven side effects in study after study over the past few decades as you will see in the next section. On the other hand, research is mounting clearly demonstrating not only the efficacy of BHRT but the safety as well. In fact, Dr. Kent Holtorf published an article in the January 2009 issue of *Postgraduate Medicine*. He cited 196 research studies and commented, "Physiological data and clinical outcomes demonstrate that bioidentical hormones are associated with lower risks, including the risk of breast cancer, cardiovascular disease, and are more efficacious than their synthetic and animal derived counterparts. Until evidence is found to the contrary, bioidentical hormones remain the preferred method of hormone replacement therapy."

Readers interested in more references on the safety of BHRT please see the REFERENCES in the back of the book for this chapter. Numerous research papers compare BHRT to HRT, specifically synthetic progesterone to bioidentical progesterone. Every single one demonstrates a greater safety profile or effectiveness of bioidentical progesterone in all categories from heart health, breast cancer, mood, PMS, menopausal symptoms and brain protection.

"When you stop taking hormone replacement therapy you lose the benefits that hormones provide almost immediately."

Smith, P., *HRT: The Answers*. 2003; Healthy Living Books, Inc., p. 9.

Option 2

Traditional Hormone Replacement Therapy (HRT)/Estrogen Replacement Therapy (ERT)

As you probably know, HRT consists of a combination of some form of estrogen with some form of progesterone. Usually the estrogen is either a synthetic estrogen or equine (horse) estrogen. Premarin®, for instance, takes its name from **preg**nant **mar**es' **uri**ne. The progesterone is usually medroxyprogesterone acetate (MPA) or some other synthetic progesterone. Synthetic progesterone is referred to as progestin. One of the most popular brands of HRT is called Prempro®. It is the combination of Premarin® derived from pregnant mare's urine and a synthetic progesterone called medroxyprogesterone acetate. So what? Estrogen is estrogen and progesterone is progesterone, right? Most unfortunately, no! Animal-derived and synthetic hormones differ greatly from endogenous (internally produced) human hormones; therein lies the problem. I will say more about this problem later. I cannot emphasize enough that synthetic and animal-derived hormones are not the same as human or bio-identical hormones.

Doctors normally prescribe simple ERT, which is estrogen-only therapy (either bio-identical or synthetic), for women whose ovaries have been removed during a hysterectomy on the theory that a woman without a uterus no longer needs progesterone to protect her from uterine cancer. However, it is now clear that progesterone has other important functions as well so that *no one* should take estrogen without progesterone. If you are taking ERT, *please* see

Chapter 3 for more information. To simplify our discussion, we will lump HRT/ERT together and use the term HRT.

More About:

HRT
According to the Women's Health Initiative study, women on Prempro have:
- *41% increased rate of stroke*
- *Double the rate of blood clots*
- *26% increase in breast cancer*
- *22% increase in heart disease*

According to the Heart and Estrogen / Progestin Replacement Study Follow Up (HERS II), women on estrogen with progestin have:
- *Increased risk of heart attacks*
- *Increased risk of blood clots in the legs and lungs*
- *Increased risk of gall bladder disease*

The Journal of the American Medical Association reported in March of 2008 women taking HRT faced a small increased risk for cancer for more than two years after they stopped taking the HRT medication.

History of HRT

For a number of decades now, traditional medicine has recognized that sex hormone deficiencies need correcting. Premarin®, mentioned above, was introduced in 1949, but it wasn't until 1966 that doctors began widely prescribing it. That was the year when Dr. Robert Wilson published his book *Feminine Forever*. With sponsorship by the manufacturer of Premarin®, the popular women's magazines of the day promoted the book in which Dr. Wilson claimed that women who took Premarin would stay "young, attractive, and sexually active," while women who didn't would see their breasts and genitalia shrivel and would become dull, unattractive, and hard to live with. It presented women in those days with an easy choice: look like Marilyn Monroe on Premarin® or become an old hag without it. Though the book presented no evidence to back up these claims, many doctors immediately began prescribing Premarin® for any woman who complained of any symptoms that might possibly be connected with menopause. Since they didn't even bother checking the woman's hormone levels to see how much, if any, estrogen she needed, millions of women were overdosed with estrogen. Eventually realizing that estrogen without (synthetic) progesterone, called unopposed estrogen, was causing uterine cancer, doctors began prescribing a combination of estrogen and synthetic progesterone to prevent uterine cancer.

Again, if you are taking unopposed estrogen because you've had a hysterectomy and are, therefore, not at risk for uterine cancer, please see Chapter 3 to learn why you still really need progesterone to protect you from other health problems.

This is as good a place as any to explain why the major drug manufacturers make their synthetic forms of estrogen and progesterone slightly different from endogenous estrogen and progesterone. Naturally occurring substances are not patentable and therefore not terribly profitable. But the manufacturers *can* produce and patent a form that differs slightly from the naturally occurring one, thereby boosting their potential profit. In fact, together Premarin® and Prempro (a combination of Premarin® and synthetic progesterone) used to generate over $2 billion a year for manufacturer Wyeth Pharmaceuticals.

For several decades doctors solved the problem of menopause by prescribing these synthetic or animal-derived hormones until research data began to reveal that they were significantly increasing the number of cases of lethal diseases like cancer and stroke. These revelations have left many in the medical profession—as well as menopausal women—stunned, not knowing how to relieve the mild to debilitating symptoms of menopause without causing much worse problems down the road. Let's examine these revelations about the dangers of traditional HRT.

More About:

The Side Effects of Prempro

Side effects of Prempro, as listed in the Physician's Desk Reference: May increase risk of cardiovascular events such as heart attacks or stroke, venous thrombosis, breast/endometrial cancer, and gallbladder disease. May also lead to hypercalcemia with breast cancer and bone metastases. Retinal vascular thrombosis reported. May elevate blood pressure, plasma triglycerides, may lead to increased thyroid binding globulin levels. May cause fluid retention or increased risk of ovarian cancer. May exacerbate endometriosis, asthma, diabetes, epilepsy or migraines. Adverse reactions include abdominal pain, back pain, headache, infection, arthralgia, leg cramps, breast pain, vaginal hemorrhage or vaginitis.

HRT Disadvantages:

First, let's look at the results of the $800 million Women's Health Initiative (WHI) research study of Prempro®. As I mentioned earlier, Prempro® is a combination of conjugated equine estrogen (Premarin®) and progestin, synthetic progesterone. This study began in 1993 with 16,608 women between the ages of fifty and seventy-nine, 30-35% of whom dropped out of the study early because of side effects or fear of side effects. The researchers themselves halted the study three years early because of alarming preliminary results.

What were they alarmed about? They discovered that women taking Prempro® had a 26% higher risk of breast cancer, a 23% higher risk of heart disease, a 38% higher risk of stroke, and a 100% higher risk of blood clots than did those in the control group. The *Journal of the American Medical Association*'s analysis of the research data showed that the breast cancers diagnosed in the study subjects on Prempro® tended to be diagnosed at more advanced stages than the breast cancers diagnosed in the women in the control group, and another article in the *Journal of the American Medical Association reported* women on Prempro® had a 56% higher risk of ovarian cancer than those in the control group. Follow-up findings also showed a higher risk of dementia and a 94% higher rate of abnormal mammograms after the first year of Prempro® usage.

In addition to these really scary side effects, women on HRT often experience many other side effects like weight gain, depression, irritability, headaches, insomnia, bloating, and gall bladder problems.

Was there any good news from this study? Not much. Improvements in quality of sleep, emotional health, and sexual satisfaction were not statistically significant, while bone density did increase and the risk of colon cancer was reduced.

How did the makers of Prempro® react to all this news? Did they immediately yank the product off the market pending further study? Did they stop selling a product that appears to be dangerous? No. Instead, they have assured the public that the increase in individual risk is "relatively small." Worse still, Wyeth Pharmaceuticals has petitioned the FDA to ban bioidentical hormones.

Sadly, a relatively small increase in risk for each individual can mean 4,200 additional cases of breast cancer, 4,800 cases of heart disease, and 10,800 strokes. Some experts have multiplied the numbers of expected cases over a decade and concluded that about 40,000 women will have been harmed by this form of HRT. Only God knows the sum of tragedies that have occurred and will occur. After all, these aren't just numbers. These women are someone's mommy, someone's soul mate, someone's precious daughter. It's heart-wrenching to say the least, and it is completely unnecessary. This study, Women's Health Initiative, was just one of many research studies that demonstrated the dangers of traditional HRT.

We've seen that HRT doesn't usually consist of hormones biologically identical to those our bodies produce; instead, it uses synthetic and animal-derived hormones (we'll call them non-bioidentical). Since non-bioidentical hormones differ in molecular structure from those the human body produces, it's not surprising that they *do not* function exactly like endogenous human hormones. Nor do our bodies process them the same way. These non-bioidentical hormones are similar enough to mimic some of the activities of the human hormones they are replacing but only in a clumsy way. While they perform some of the vital functions of endogenous hormones, they can cause problems the human-produced hormones do not.

For one thing, they are hard to metabolize. Our bodies metabolize endogenous and bioidentical hormones easily and efficiently, but we can't say the same for non-bioidentical hormones. For instance, in the human body metabolites (the by-products of metabolism) of conjugated equine estrogen (derived from horse urine) are stronger than the parent compound and can be converted into carcinogens right in breast tissue. Metabolites from conjugated equine estrogen can stay in the body up to thirteen weeks while the body clears human estrogen in a few hours. And medroxyprogesterone acetate (MPA, a synthetic progesterone known as Provera) contains extra atoms in unusual positions on the molecule that inhibit metabolism and so prolong its activity in the body.

Another difference between endogenous and bioidentical hormones and non-bioidentical hormones is in their relative binding affinity (RBA). A hormone molecule's RBA is its ability to bind with receptor sites in various cells throughout the body. Normally a hormone molecule floats along in the bloodstream until it reaches a cell that has receptor sites designed specifically for that hormone to attach itself to. Once attached, it is able to perform whatever chemical activity it is supposed to perform in that cell. For example, a cell in the uterine lining has receptor sites for progesterone. When a molecule of progesterone reaches the receptor site, it should attach itself and begin to prime the endometrial cell, preparing it to nourish any fertilized egg that might attach to the endometrium. So you can see that the fact that MPA has an RBA of just 6% compared to endogenous progesterone's 100% RBA means that while 100% of the natural progesterone molecules that encounter endometrial cell receptor sites will attach themselves properly, only 6% of MPA molecules do so. Obviously, Provera (synthetic progesterone) can't possibly function as well as endogenous progesterone.

The opposite problem can occur as well. Sometimes the non-bioidentical hormone molecule tends to bind too tightly to a receptor site, causing improper metabolism or simply preventing the receptors from receiving endogenous hormones. That is, because the non-bioidentical hormone molecule is occupying the receptor site but is unable to perform its function; endogenous hormone molecules are unable to attach themselves to that site. It is like having a tiny little compact car in your garage so you cannot get your Cadillac in it. Even worse, non-bioidentical progestins are able to bind to other receptors, like glucocorticoid, androgen, and mineralocorticoid receptors (intended for testosterone and cortisol to bind to), which may explain the wide range of adverse side effects many women experience while taking synthetic progestins.

Not surprisingly, the dysfunction of these non-bioidentical hormones can cause all sorts of side effects not caused by endogenous or bioidentical hormones. In fact, women taking Provera almost always suffer some side effects. And since Premarin® is actually toxic to DNA, it's not too astonishing that it causes side effects too. Maybe this explains why 80% of women discontinue HRT within one year.

More About:

Side Effects of Provera (MPA), A Common Synthetic Progestin

Decreased glucose tolerance, gastric regurgitation, depression, anxiety, fluid retention, adverse effects on lipids, insomnia, headache, nervousness, acne, dizziness, facial hair, loss of scalp hair, weight gain, rash or itch, breast tenderness, or nipple discharge. It is also believed to increase the risk of coronary heart disease and blood clots.

Commonly Prescribed Hormones Chart

It is important to note, however, that not all traditional HRT is non-bioidentical. Some commonly used hormones, such as estrogen patches, are actually bioidentical, but not all. Refer to chart below.

Product Name	*Bioidentical*
Premarin	no
Cenestin	no
Ortho-Est	Estrogen-yes Progesterone-no
Ogen	no
Menest	no
Prempro	no
FemHRT	no
Ortho-Prefest	no
Activella	Estrogen-yes Progesterone-no
Premphase	no
Provera	no
Cycrin	no
Curretab	no
Amen	no
Aygestin	no
Megace	no
ClimaraPro	Estrogen-yes Progesterone-no

CombiPatch	Estrogen-yes Progesterone-no
Evista	no
Estratest	no
Methytest	no
Estrogel	yes
Estrasorb	yes
Elestrin	yes
**Biest Transdermal or Oral	yes
**Triest Transdermal or Oral	yes
Gynodiol	yes
Estrace	yes
Estradiol	yes
**Estriol Transdermal or Oral	yes
Prometrium	yes
**Progesterone Transdermal or Oral	yes
Alora	yes
Climara	yes
Esclim	yes
Estraderm	yes
Menostar	yes
Vivelle Dot	yes
**Testosterone	yes
Crinone	yes
Procheive	yes
Vagifem	yes
Estring	yes

Femring	*
Estradiol cypionate	*
Estradiol valerate	*
Hydroxyprogesterone caproate	*
Testosterone cypionate	*
DepoTestadiol	*

*Conditional-these products are bioidentical, but are chemically bonded to other substances.
** **Compounded Hormones**

Oral Contraceptives – The Pill

Women from teens to perimenopausal age are often given the pill to manage symptoms related to hormone imbalance. While it is true that the pill can help alleviate symptoms, it does not correct the underlying hormone imbalances. The pill works by blocking Follicle Stimulating Hormone (FSH) and Luteinizing Hormone (LH). This in turn reduces the production of natural estrogen, progesterone and testosterone. For women who might have been making excessive amounts of estrogen or testosterone this might seem to be a relief. For others, reduced amounts of hormones create symptoms of low estrogen or testosterone. This could trigger symptoms such as low libido, weight gain, bone loss and vaginal dryness.

It is very important to consider the fact that since the pill blocks ovulation, progesterone is not made, leaving women on the pill progesterone deficient. This is a strong point to consider because as you will see in Chapter 3, the roles and properties of progesterone are so vital to a woman's health, especially in regard to protecting the breast tissue.

Unlike the human hormones estrogen and testosterone, the hormones in the pill are not bound to any Sex Hormone Binding Globulin in the body so the synthetic hormones are widely available to impart their effects. (Sex Hormone Binding Globulin is a protein made by the liver that binds to some hormones making them less available to the body.) The synthetic hormones in the pill can act on different hormone receptors in the body. You see, human estrogen acts on estrogen receptors, human testosterone acts on testosterone receptors and so on. The synthetic hormones in the pill can act on testosterone receptors causing symptoms of excessive levels and creating a testosterone deficiency at the same time. The synthetic progesterone in the pill can act like cortisol and suppress normal adrenal hormone activity. The pill can also increase Thyroid Binding Globulin (a binding protein that binds to thyroid hormones making less available) and impair thyroid hormone function leading to symptoms related to hypothyroidism. And sometimes the ovaries don't bounce back to normal hormone production once the pill is discontinued. All in all, the pill might be a quick fix for some symptoms; but it can create hormone imbalances and cause problems in the long run.

Option 3

OTC

Many women, wishing to avoid synthetic and animal-derived hormones, treat themselves with OTC phytoestrogens (estrogenic substances that come from plants). Many medical and nutrition practitioners recommend them as well.

More about:

Phytoestrogens

Phytoestrogens are "estrogen-like" chemicals found in more than three hundred plant foods. Soybeans have some of the highest levels of phytoestrogens and have been studied

*the most. There are three chemical classes: the isoflavonoids,
the lignans, or the coumestans.*

In distinguishing between bioidentical hormones and phytoestrogens, it all comes back to the shape of the molecule. These plant estrogens have similar molecular structures, but they're not identical to human hormones. Essentially, they can activate the estrogen receptor but are much, much weaker than the real human or bioidentical estrogen.

Many women with low estrogen symptoms and women with estrogen levels on the low side of normal on their hormone test respond very well to OTC products like phytoestrogens from soy isoflavones or black cohosh, which is not technically a phytoestrogen. Phytoestrogens, in some cases, may resolve low estrogen symptoms like hot flashes.

But I have to suggest that you approach OTC remedies with caution because while they do help many women, they can sometimes cause other hormones to become imbalanced. For instance, many phytoestrogens contain something called aromatase inhibitors. Basically aromatase is the enzyme that converts testosterone in our bodies into estrogen. Whether this conversion is good or bad depends on your current hormone levels, so you have to be careful and be properly monitored with saliva hormone testing.

Another possible problem with phytoestrogens is that they can actually suppress production of endogenous estrogen, causing your estrogen levels to drop. Again, depending on your hormone levels, it may or may not be appropriate. But because phytoestrogen molecules fit in human estrogen receptors, the phytoestrogens themselves can function as estrogen and activate estrogen-related genes. Therefore, it is possible for them to simultaneously lower estrogen levels and cause symptoms of estrogen dominance, and they may or may not be effective in reducing hot flashes. Adding to the confusion, it is impossible to measure the level of phytoestrogens in the body. And some experts question whether OTC phytoestrogens protect against such hormone deficiency-related conditions as bone density loss, memory loss, and cholesterol problems.

Black Cohosh does seem to show much promise for symptom relief but actually works by a different mechanism than by activating the estrogen receptor. It appears to work by the same mechanism that allows many doctors to prescribe anti-depressants (SSRIs-Selective Serotonin Reuptake Inhibitors) for hot flashes. Even more encouraging, recent animal and in vitro research indicates that black cohosh can stop the progression of a human breast cancer cell line.

While many studies do report the effectiveness of phytoestrogens for the management of menopausal symptoms, there is controversy regarding the use of isoflavones from soy, as recent studies now question the safety of phytoestrogens in women with or at high risk for hormonal cancers.

One study conducted over a five year period showed that phytoestrogen supplementation increases the risk of developing endometrial hyperplasia, or thickening of the uterine lining, elevating the risk of endometrial cancer. I have to wonder whether adding progesterone to the phytoestrogen could prevent the hyperplasia.

There is also the question about whether women who have had breast cancer or who are at high risk for it should use phytoestrogen. As I understand it, research is inconclusive, yet this question is concerning to me. Animal studies have shown that genistein in soy increased the proliferation (multiplication) of estrogen-dependent human breast cancer cells. Studies have also shown that soy protein isolate stimulates breast tissue in 30% of pre-menopausal women. Additional research has found that the use of soy isoflavones increased secretion of breast fluid and elevated estrogen levels.

Note: If you are taking Tamoxifen for breast cancer, genistein was shown to interfere or block the effectiveness of the drug.

There is also concern that large amounts of soy can inhibit thyroid function. For this reason, a general recommendation is not to take excessive amounts and to consult your physician before taking it.

I am not saying you definitely shouldn't use phytoestrogens, but I am alerting you to possible problems. People tend to think that since they come from plants they must be universally good for you or at least harmless. Once again, it comes down to proper testing and monitoring.

On a positive note, there is significant mounting research on the benefits of phytoestrogens. Again, common forms are soy, pomegranate, flax seed, black cohosh and red clover. One recent example of this encouraging data is the report on ground flax seed. The summer 2007 issue of the *Journal of the Society for Integrative Oncology* reported a study conducted at the Mayo Clinic which found that consuming forty grams of crushed/ground flaxseed reduced hot flashes; the frequency was cut in half and the overall "hot flash score" had diminished by an average of 57%. The women also reported improved mood, reduced joint or muscle pain, fewer chills and less sweating. In recent trials, flax has been shown to help decrease the risk of breast cancer. The seeds are also a source of omega-3 fatty acids and fiber. The lignans in flax seeds are very breast protective.

Option 4

Letting Nature Take Its Course

There are many reasons why women choose to let nature take its course without interference. Women who sail through their repro-ductive years and menopause with little discomfort of any kind often don't even consider interfering. But if you're reading this book, chances are your seas are a bit rough or maybe downright stormy. Many women in this situation still choose to do nothing, viewing their hormonal suffering as simply their lot in life to be endured-just part of being a woman. If generations of women have suffered such miseries, why should they escape? Well for one thing, it's very likely that because of diet and environmental factors hor-monal imbalances are much more common today than in the past. Second, a pretty large chunk of human suffering has been eradicated in our era simply because of advances in knowledge and technology. These advances have, in turn, caused us trouble our forebears didn't have to contend with in regard to health, so we might as well take the good along with the bad.

And then there's the "tough guy" attitude that I "should" be woman enough to take the suffering. Well, OK if you want. And some women hesitate to get help because money is an issue. That reasoning is very understandable, but it can be kind of like dental work-maybe spend some money now or spend a lot of money and endure a lot of pain later. So, I guess we could say that the advantage of doing nothing is the immediate saving of time and money, but the disadvantages are unnecessary suffering, possibly a severe strain on your career, marriage, and other relationships, and possibly long-term, serious adverse effects on your health. Whether your reasons for gritting your teeth are spiritual, emotional, or financial, there are also medically sound reasons for correcting hormone imbalances. Cancer, heart disease, osteoporosis, or other serious health problems can result from long-term hormone imbalances.

In conclusion, hormone imbalances are complex, requiring a comprehensive approach to restoring balance and protecting against hormone related diseases. BHRT is a comprehensive modality that can greatly improve your health and quality of life. For me personally and for countless others, it is the only option, especially when combined with a good complement of supplements.

Chapter 3

WHAT ARE HORMONES ANYWAY?

This chapter is for those interested in a deeper understanding of the science of hormones and the common causes of hormone imbalance. It also delves into symptoms of deficiency and excessive levels of estrogen, progesterone, and testosterone. It then explains the roles and function of these three key reproductive hormones.

Before discussing hormone imbalances, we need to talk about what hormones are and how they work. The word *hormone* comes from the Greek word for stimulate, excite, stir up, impulse, and assault; it is related to arouse. Hormones certainly can do all of these, right? Hormones are chemical messengers synthesized (produced) in various glands and secreted into the blood stream where they travel until they encounter special hormone receptor sites on various cells.

You can think of a hormone molecule as a car key and the receptor site as a car's ignition. When the hormone "key" fits into the receptor site "ignition" and turns, the cell starts performing whatever vital function the hormone directs. Of course, different hormones perform different functions, and the same hormone can perform a variety of roles, depending on the type of cell it encounters. For example, estrogen performs one function in brain cells, another in muscle cells, and yet another in breast tissue.

More About:

How Hormones Work:

Hormones go from the blood → to the specific cell membranes of the target tissue with specific receptors for the specific hormone → to the cell nucleus → then interact with the DNA → to produce RNA → once this action terminates, the hormone leaves or is metabolized. Did you know that hormones interact with your DNA, the entire foundation of your metabolism?

This process is complicated by the fact that hormones travel through the bloodstream in one of two states: bound or free. While free hormones can enter a cell's receptor sites as described above, bound hormones cannot because bound hormones are covered by a protein coat. It's as if the hormone "key" is covered with a glove or mitten that prevents it from fitting into the receptor site "ignition." It is like your car keys in your purse, they certainly cannot be put into the ignition. Sex hormone-binding globulin (SHBG) is the protein coat that binds itself to estrogen, testosterone, and a testosterone metabolite called dihydrotestosterone (DHT). Cortisol binding globulin (CBG) binds to progesterone and cortisol. These binding proteins are there to help clear hormones from the body. Approximately 1 to 5% of the hormones are "free" or unbound to a binding protein, compared to 95 to 99% that are protein bound. The higher the levels of various hormone binding proteins in your bloodstream, the more hormone molecules will be bound, lowering the level of functional hormones in your bloodstream. So what's the point? When you have your hormones tested, make very sure that your health care practitioner orders tests that measure levels of *free* hormones rather than simply the total amount of each hormone. (Please see hormone testing in Chapter 4.)

More About:

Hormones

Hormone: A naturally occurring substance secreted by specialized cells such as in glands that affect the metabolism or action on other cells. Hormones typically act on cells that have receptors for the hormone. Hormones may be hydrophilic (more water soluble), such as insulin, or lipophilic (fat soluble) like the sex hormones. Water soluble hormones act on receptors on the cell surface while fat soluble hormones act on receptors in the cells.

The Normal Menstrual Cycle

Let's take a minute to refresh our memories about the normal menstrual cycle. The first day of flow is considered Day One, and it is on Day One that estrogen, progesterone, and testosterone are at their lowest levels. The pituitary gland secretes follicle-stimulating hormone (FSH) to stimulate the ovaries to produce estrogen and prepare an egg for ovulation. On about Day Seven, the estrogen level begins to rise, causing the lining of the uterus (endometrium) to begin thickening. Meanwhile, one or more eggs begin to develop in a follicle in the ovary. During this first two weeks of the cycle, called the follicular phase, estrogen is the dominant hormone. Ovulation occurs about fourteen days into the cycle when the follicle ruptures, releasing the egg into the fallopian tube, whence it travels to the uterus. What's left of the ruptured follicle is called the corpus luteum (Latin for "yellow body" because it happens to be yellow), which begins producing progesterone. The progesterone level rises to high levels and is the dominant hormone throughout the second half (luteal phase) of the cycle. The function of progesterone is to prime or mature the endometrial cells to nurture any embryo that arrives. If no embryo attaches to the uterine lining, estrogen and progesterone levels drop on about Day Twenty-six, triggering the shedding of the endometrial lining beginning on about Day Twenty-eight and starting the cycle all over again. When hormones flow in nice balance, there are no symptoms such as what may occur pre-menstrually.

Menstrual Cycle Hormone Levels

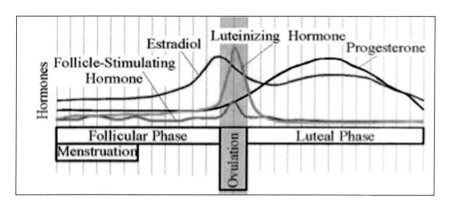

One **crucial** fact to note here: if a woman does not ovulate, she produces negligible amounts of progesterone, leaving her progesterone deficient and in an estrogen dominant state all month long. Since birth control pills block ovulation, they block virtually all progesterone production. Birth control pills do contain a synthetic form of progesterone, but as we have seen elsewhere in this book, it's a very poor substitute.

Reproductive Phases of a Woman's Life

Before we go further, let's define the different phases of a woman's reproductive life so we'll be clear as we go on.

Premenopause: This term simply refers to a woman's child-bearing years between the onset of her first menstrual period and the cessation of cycles.

Perimenopause: From *peri*, meaning "around," this term defines the period of up to ten years prior to menopause during which estrogen levels tend to fluctuate, often making a woman feel like she's on an emotional roller coaster and causing cycles to become irregular. Progesterone levels tend to be low during perimenopause.

Menopause: Women are officially in menopause after twelve consecutive months without a menstrual period. Recall that before menopause the pituitary gland secretes follicle-stimulating hormone (FSH) each month to stimulate the ovaries to produce estrogen and prepare an egg for ovulation. At menopause, when the ovaries fail to accomplish these tasks, the pituitary gland secretes more FSH. FSH rises above normal levels as the pituitary continues producing FSH in a futile effort to stimulate the ovaries. Levels of luteinizing hormone (LH) and estrogen usually remain normal or slightly higher for about a year until follicle failure occurs.

Postmenopause: The time following menopause defined by the permanent cessation of the menstrual cycles. Postmenopausal levels of hormones are typically low, possibly deficient, and do not fluctuate on a monthly basis as during the reproductive years.

More About:

Testing for Menopause

Your doctor can use a blood test to measure the level of Follicle Stimulating Hormone (FSH) to check your menopausal status. Blood levels of FSH higher than twenty three may indicate menopause. There are two things to remember about this menopause test. First of all, the FSH level can periodically go up and down during perimenopause. Therefore, it is not necessarily a definitive test. Secondly, an FSH test does not reveal your level of estrogen, progesterone, or testosterone.

What Most Women Experience

Sex hormone levels decline with age, and there's just no way around it. No drug, herb, or therapy will prevent it, and that's alright-God designed it that way. Otherwise, we would have menstrual cycles all our lives. But when hormones decline too much or behave erratically, the results can be unpleasant and even dangerous. Women typically begin to experience symptoms of progesterone deficiency in their mid-thirties. Women may also have high levels of cortisol, under-active thyroids, and unstable blood sugar. (We'll discuss cortisol, thyroid hormones, and blood sugar problems in Chapter 5.) While estrogen levels usually remain normal until later, progesterone begins to fall, often dropping by as much as 75% by the time menopause occurs. As progesterone levels drop, the nice equilibrium between estrogen and progesterone begins to break down. Research suggests that by the age of thirty-five, half of all women are progesterone deficient. Because estrogen and progesterone are meant to be in balance with each other, progesterone deficiency often causes a syndrome called estrogen dominance.

More About:

Estrogen Dominance

Estrogen Dominance occurs when there is not enough progesterone to balance the level of estrogen. Some experts believe that there should be one hundred to five hundred times more progesterone than estrogen. Relative progesterone-to-estrogen deficiency can contribute to such symptoms as breast pain or cysts, uterine fibroids, PMS, fluid retention, and heavy periods. Estrogen dominance can occur with elevated estrogen, normal levels of estrogen, or estrogen deficiency. It is essentially progesterone deficiency. Saliva hormone testing shows estrogen dominance with the Pg/E2 ratio. That is called progesterone-to-estradiol ratio.

The Most Common Causes of Hormone Imbalances

1. Age: Normal age-related decline in hormone levels is the most common cause of hormone imbalances and deficiencies. Levels of estrogen, progesterone, and testosterone all decline as we grow older.

Age –Related Decline of Hormones

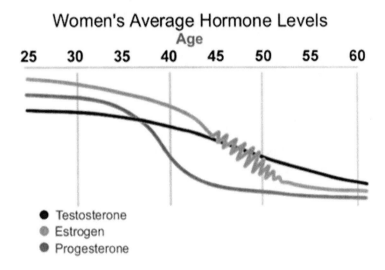

As seen in the graph, progesterone typically begins to decline by the mid-thirties, estrogen fluctuates and declines on average in the forties, and testosterone makes a gradual decline.

2. Stress: Stress is also a major culprit in hormone problems. It affects the adrenal glands in such a way that the levels of stress hormones, in this case, DHEA and Cortisol, are initially elevated. This situation can, in turn, create excessive levels of estrogen or testosterone. Eventually, long term chronic stress can lower DHEA levels, and since DHEA is a major source of testosterone for women, testosterone levels can drop as a result. DHEA contributes to about 40% of the total testosterone synthesis as well as 40% of the estradiol (estrogen) production. And stress has a very interesting effect on progesterone. Because your body uses progesterone to block cortisol at the cortisol receptor sites, high levels of cortisol can rapidly deplete progesterone. Further, elevated cortisol triggers symptoms of just about every type of hormone imbalance and low cortisol has its own effects on the other hormones. Paradoxically, low estrogen (estradiol) causes increased Cortisol Binding Protein, which binds up cortisol, making less available. This is all very complicated; therefore, I have dedicated an entire section in Chapter 5 to explain this relationship with cortisol in greater detail. For now, take it from me, stress does indeed cause hormone imbalance.

3. Weight Gain: Weight gain affects hormone levels by increasing the level of aromatase. Aromatase is an enzyme that converts testosterone into estrogen in a process called, not surprisingly, aromatization. Since fat contains higher levels of aromatase than other tissues, fat produces more estrogen. Since excess estrogen encourages weight gain, you can see how easy it is to end up in a vicious cycle. So, in some cases, the more weight you gain, the more estrogen the extra fat produces. The excess estrogen, coupled with low progesterone, encourages fat formation, and women get caught in a miserable spiral. However, because we are all unique and bio-chemically different, do not assume that because you have extra weight you make plenty of estrogen. I have seen countless women with a few extra pounds who have extremely low estrogen levels. By the way, low estrogen causes weight gain. Are you getting the point that all of the hormones must be in balance to maintain your waistline?

4. Diet: Sometimes hormone imbalances result from poor diet and nutritional deficiencies. Zinc deficiency, for example, can lower levels of Sex Hormone Binding Globulin, SHBG. This is a binding protein made by the liver which can bind to estrogen, testosterone or DHEA. The lower the level of SHBG, the higher the levels of free estrogen and testosterone will be. High fat, low fiber diets, elevated stress hormone, cortisol, weight gain and alcohol consumption can decrease SHBG and in turn throw hormones out of balance. And sugars and refined starches impair liver function, which can also cause hormonal problems because your liver is vital to hormone metabolism. Also, excessive carbohydrates cause blood sugar and insulin imbalance, which, in turn, can negatively affect the other hormones.

5. Failure to Ovulate: Since it's the egg follicle that ultimately pro-duces progesterone, failure to ovulate is a very common cause of progesterone shortage. Women commonly begin to skip ovulation frequently as they move into their late thirties and forties.

6. Ovarian Dysfunction: Hormone imbalances can also result when the ovaries simply produce too much or too little estrogen, proges-terone, or testosterone for various reasons. For example, the ovaries of women with polycystic ovarian syndrome (PCOS) overproduce testosterone and DHEA goes up. Some experts are beginning to sus-pect that women are just not producing as much progesterone as they did decades ago. It is also possible that exposure of unborn baby girls to xenoestrogens (chemical estrogens in the environment) affects their ovarian function. These dangerous and toxic synthetic estrogens can lead to follicular failure in adulthood, though the mechanism by which it might occur is not understood.

7. Other Glandular Dysfunctions: Dysfunctions of other glands, such as the thyroid and adrenals, can cause sex hormone imbalances. Please see Chapter 5 on thyroid hormones and adrenal hormones.

8. Non-bioidentical Hormones: Synthetic or animal-derived hormones, like those in oral contraceptives and traditional HRT, can also cause hormone imbalance. For instance, birth control pills block ovulation. Without ovulation, there is no endogenous progesterone production. The lack of progesterone can cause estrogen dominance. As I've said before, the synthetic progesterone birth control pills provide does not perform the same way as endogenous progesterone. Synthetic hormones, whether from HRT or oral contraceptive, fail to give complete messages to create a normal or balanced hormone response.

Essentially, synthetic hormones in birth control pills or patches lower the production of estrogen, progesterone, and testosterone. Also, the synthetic hormones in birth control pills interfere with cortisol and increase the risk of insulin resistance, which is the reason many women gain weight around the waist when taking the pill. There are other reasons why the synthetic hormones in the pill throw hormones out of balance too. The synthetic hormones will act on several different receptors. For example, the synthetic progesterone can also act on androgen receptors, causing symptoms of elevated androgens like testosterone, but it actually lowers testosterone production.

You see, while taking the pill, Sex Hormone Binding Globulin (SHBG) production increases; this protein binds up testosterone and estrogen, making less available to tissues. This can cause low testosterone or estrogen issues such as low libido, bone loss, or vaginal dryness to name a few. Moreover, the pill acts on the pituitary gland in the brain, shutting down Follicle Stimulating Hormone and Luteinizing Hormone. This is why it sometimes takes a while for cycles to resume with normalcy when a woman stops taking the pill. Sadly, sometimes normal ovarian function does not resume.

Another interesting point is that real hormones (estrogen, progesterone, and testosterone) only see and act on their own receptors. Human and bioidentical progesterone, for example, only act on the progesterone receptor, not on the cortisol receptor like the synthetic version. If all of this seems confusing, rest assured that it will all make more sense as we delve deeper into each of these hormones and how they relate.

The non-bioidentical hormones in traditional HRT and ERT only mimic endogenous hormones, and they often trigger side effects instead of truly correcting the hormone imbalances and the problems associated with those imbalances they're supposed to fix. Traditional HRT, taken orally, lowers testosterone levels too, leaving women at risk of low testosterone symptoms. Testosterone deficiency can lead to loss of bone. Since bone loss is something HRT is supposed to prevent, the actual outcome may not necessarily offer optimal bone protection. Even more, oral HRT triggers the binding of thyroid hormones, often causing functional hypothyroidism. You can see how non-bioidentical hormones can cause more problems than they supposedly prevent.

9. Xenoestrogens: Xenoestrogens and other endocrine disrupters are synthetic chemicals with molecular structures similar to those of estrogens. Produced by industrial, agricultural, and chemical companies from a variety of sources, they are found in air, water, and food. They're even similar enough that molecules of these chemicals fit into estrogen receptors. Many researchers are beginning to suspect that these substances are causing hormonal imbalances. The synthetic estrogens used to fatten cattle also activate estrogen receptors, causing estrogen dominance in women and also in men, possibly having a negative effect on the prostate.

More About:

Causes of Hormone Imbalance as Explained by Dr. Joseph Narrins, OB/GYN, Gaffney, SC:
- *Guy*necologists
- *Men*strual cycles
- *His*terectomies
- Pre*men*strual syndrome
- *Men*opause
- *Men*tal problems

Now that we understand how hormones work in general and what can cause imbalances, let's look at what each specific hormone we're talking about actually *does*. Then it'll be easy to see why it's so important to have enough of each hormone and the right balance among hormones for a perfect hormone makeover. Refer back to each section as necessary, especially when you get hormone test results back.

Progesterone Deficiency

Let's start with progesterone since progesterone is the first hormone that begins to decline. As mentioned earlier, progesterone deficiency can start in the mid-thirties and continue declining by as much as 75% by the time we reach menopause.

More About:

Causes of Progesterone Deficiency

- *Impaired or reduced ovarian production*
- *Low levels of luteinizing hormone (LH)*
- *Excess levels of prolactin*
- *Chronic stress*
- *Antidepressants*
- *Dietary: excessive sugar or saturated fat*
- *Nutrient deficiencies: A, B6, C, Zinc*
- *Thyroid Problems*

First, as you'd expect, progesterone deficiency causes menstrual problems, like irregular or shorter time between cycles, and PMS symptoms, like fluid retention, bloating, breast pain, irritability,

78

and carbohydrate cravings. Insufficient progesterone can also cause cramps, spotting between periods, heavy bleeding, blood clots, uterine fibroids, and endometriosis. It can even cause infertility and miscarriage. Progesterone deficiency can trigger endocrine problems such as functional hypothyroidism (symptoms of low thyroid with normal lab values). Therefore, low body temperature, slow metabolism, weight gain, and hair loss may all be present. Progesterone deficiency can affect blood sugar balance, trigger headaches, worsen allergies and sinusitis, and increase wrinkling of the skin. It can also lead to the much more serious problems of bone loss, fibrocystic breast disease, and breast cancer.

Symptoms and Conditions of Progesterone Deficiency:

General Physical Symptoms or Related Conditions:
- *Weight gain*
- *Fluid retention*
- *Low body temperature*
- *Hypothyroidism (under-activity of the thyroid gland)*
- *Headaches*
- *Pain and inflammation*
- *Allergies/sinusitis*
- *Insomnia or sleep disturbances*
- *Hair loss*
- *Bone loss*

Gynecological Symptoms or Related Conditions:
- *PMS*
- *Cramps*
- *Breast pain/benign cysts*
- *Heavy periods*
- *Irregular cycles (periods too close together)*
- *Spotting before period or break-through bleeding*
- *Fibroids*
- *Endometriosis*
- *Infertility*
- *Miscarriage*
- *Luteal phase deficiency (a common cause of infertility)*

Emotional Symptoms or Related Conditions:
- *Depression*
- *Anxiety*
- *Irritability*
- *Mood swings*
- *Tendency to be stressed easily*

What Progesterone Does for You

When we think of women's hormones, we usually think first of estrogen, but progesterone is just as important. In fact, it's hard to overstate its importance. There are progesterone receptor sites in every cell of your body, so progesterone affects virtually all of your cells. Progesterone has multiple non-reproductive roles including functions in the central nervous system to regulate cognition, mood, inflammation, mitochondrial function, neurogenesis and regeneration (the formation and development of nerve cells), myelination (formation of the insulation around nerves) and recovery from brain injury. It must be vital to your health, right?

If you're reading this book, chances are you are progesterone-deficient. How do I know you are most likely progesterone deficient? Progesterone deficiency typically occurs at least by age thirty-five when the follicles begin to lose their ability to produce normal levels of progesterone. While you may think hormone deficiency affects only your comfort and quality of life, the truth is that it can actually affect the length of your life as well. The good news is that bioidentical progesterone is widely available now without a prescription, so no woman has to be progesterone deficient; after reading this section, you won't want to be. Let's look first at where and how your body produces progesterone, and then we'll see how it affects different tissues, body systems, and processes.

As mentioned earlier, during a normal menstrual cycle, the ruptured follicle (corpus luteum) that releases the egg begins producing progesterone after ovulation. During this luteal phase, Days 14-28 of the cycle, the corpus luteum produces 4-28 mg of progesterone per day. The exact amount varies with each woman and with each day of her cycle. Interestingly enough, a woman's central and peripheral nervous systems also produce very small quantities of progesterone. The adrenal glands also produce progesterone as a precursor of cortisol. And during the second and third trimesters of pregnancy, the placenta produces massive amounts of progesterone (about 300 mg), which brings us to progesterone's role in pregnancy. Also interesting to note is that women make one hundred times more progesterone than estrogen, or at least we are supposed to do so.

Progesterone in Pregnancy

Progesterone is necessary for a fertilized egg to implant in the uterus, is essential for proper fetal brain development, and helps prevent miscarriage. During the first twelve weeks of pregnancy (before the placenta begins producing progesterone in sufficient quantities), if the mother's progesterone level is too low, the uterine lining can break down, causing miscarriage. By the second trimester, the placenta takes over production to produce the high levels required during pregnancy. By the third trimester, the placenta makes massive amounts of progesterone. Therefore, babies are exposed to very high amounts, around 300 mg. Think about that fact. Our precious, unborn babies are exposed to such extremely high levels of progesterone. That says a lot about the safety of progesterone. Though it is a sex hormone, it produces no secondary sex characteristics like estrogen, which conveys feminine properties, or testosterone, which conveys masculinizing properties.

David Zava, PhD., author of *What Your Doctor May Not Tell You about Breast Cancer*, indicates that progesterone deficiency during pregnancy may lead to improper brain development in the unborn child leading to ADD. This may occur because progesterone is essential for development of regions of the brain necessary for shuttling information, or memory.

Many practitioners report restoration of fertility with progesterone. I have personally known several patients that have been able to conceive and carry their baby full term with progesterone therapy.

Progesterone researcher Dr. Katherina Dalton, who has studied progesterone for over thirty years in England, has long held that women who use progesterone during pregnancy have babies with higher IQ's and less colic. One interesting study she published about prenatal progesterone therapy and educational attainments appeared in the *British Journal of Psychiatry*. This study compared educational attainments of thirty-four children whose mothers received prenatal progesterone with thirty-seven normal and twelve toxemic controls. Results at ages seventeen to twenty-four showed that progesterone children were more likely to continue schooling after sixteen years, a higher number left school with 'O' and 'A' level grades, and more obtained entrance to university. The best academic results were found for children whose mothers had received over five grams of progesterone for a minimum of eight weeks, with treatment beginning before week sixteen of pregnancy. Another researcher, Renish, in the journal, *The Female Patient*, from 1978 found that the use of progesterone increases a child's IQ, typically by around 35 points and produces personalities that are more "independent, individualistic, self-assured, self-sufficient and sensitive".

Progesterone also helps prepare the breasts for lactation. I personally used transdermal progesterone in three of my four pregnancies. I wish I had known to use it during my first pregnancy.

Progesterone in the Menstrual Cycle

Progesterone is also very important when pregnancy does not occur because it prevents spotting between periods and can often extend the cycle of a woman whose menstrual cycle is too short-less than twenty-eight days long. By balancing estrogen, it can prevent heavy bleeding and reduce blood clots, dramatically alleviate menstrual cramps, inhibit the growth of uterine fibroids, and curb endometriosis. *And* it is a woman's first line of defense against PMS. It can greatly alleviate bloating, irritability, carbohydrate cravings, and breast pain that occurs prior to the cycles. Dr. Joel Hargrove of Vanderbilt University published research demonstrating 90 percent success rate in treating PMS with bioidentical progesterone.

Progesterone's Relationship with Estrogen

One of the most important things to understand about progesterone is its relationship with estrogen. It balances and enhances the beneficial effects of estrogen while preventing problems excess estrogen can cause. For starters, progesterone is necessary for the creation of estrogen receptor sites in your cells, so you must have progesterone in order for estrogen to function in your body. This function is why in many women progesterone can actually alleviate estrogen deficiency symptoms like hot flashes. In fact, one study found that two-thirds of postmenopausal women actually still make enough estrogen, but when progesterone plummets with the cessation of ovulation, women may not be able to use the estrogen they *are* producing. A 1999 study published in *Obstetrics and Gynecology* found that transdermally administered progesterone alleviated hot flashes in 83% of menopausal women, and several other studies have demonstrated the effectiveness of progesterone cream on menopausal symptoms. Progesterone won't raise the level of estrogen in truly estrogen-deficient women; instead, it just enables the body to use the estrogen it has. Very often, that's all a woman needs.

Estrogen Dominance

There is a lot written about what is called "Estrogen Dominance." As I said, progesterone must balance estrogen. (There should be one hundred to five hundred times more progesterone than estrogen.) When the balance tilts in favor of estrogen, estrogen dominance results. This condition is particularly common in women in their mid-thirties through early forties when estrogen production remains high while ovulation begins to falter, thereby dramatically cutting progesterone production. Estrogen dominance causes many problems and creates several other imbalances-many fall under the category of progesterone deficiency. Simply stated, estrogen dominance is just progesterone deficiency. You see, you can have a normal estrogen level, elevated estrogen, or even low estrogen and have estrogen dominance if you do not have enough progesterone to balance the estrogen. Estrogen dominance impairs thyroid hormone conversion to its most active forms, leading to symptoms of hypothyroidism. And estrogen dominance increases the amount of Thyroid Binding Globulin, which means less thyroid hormone is available to thyroid receptors. Excessive estrogen down-regulates the androgen receptors and binds up some of the androgens in the blood, creating androgen deficiency or symptoms of low androgens. Testosterone and DHEA are both androgens and play very important roles in our health.

As we've mentioned earlier, estrogen is produced not only by the ovaries but also in fat tissue. On the other hand, the only way your body can produce appreciable quantities of progesterone is through ovulation. If ovulation is compromised, a woman will be starved for progesterone.

Progesterone as a Diuretic

Progesterone is the most powerful endogenous diuretic your body produces, and it is a potassium-sparing diuretic. This means that while many diuretics deplete your body's stores of potassium, progesterone helps your body maintain the proper sodium/potassium ratio. So, if a woman is low in progesterone, she can tend to have that dreaded premenstrual water retention.

Progesterone and Weight

Progesterone is thermogenic, which means it speeds up metabolism, so it helps women burn calories for energy instead of storing them as fat. Speaking of fat storage, proper levels of progesterone are necessary for the regulation of insulin, the fat-storage hormone. Estrogen dominance causes more frequent and rapid release of insulin, and fluctuations in estrogen and progesterone levels also stimulate insulin release. Excess insulin in the blood causes carbohydrate cravings because your body wants to raise your blood sugar level to balance the high insulin level. A proper progesterone/estrogen ratio tempers insulin release, helping normalize blood sugar levels and reducing cravings. (Please see Insulin section in Chapter 5.)

Progesterone's Role in Breast Health

Every woman needs to know the vital role proge
in protecting against breast cancer. A Johns Hopkins st
long ago as 1981, that half of all breast cancers could be prevented
by having a normal amount of progesterone. Studies have also shown
that breast cancer patients who had adequate progesterone at the time
of surgery lived longer than those who didn't. Progesterone cream has
been shown to reduce breast cell proliferation 400%, and when used
with estrogen cream, progesterone stopped the proliferatory effect of
estrogen. Even more, in tumor samples of women with breast cancer
taking progesterone, the tumors are well differentiated, quiescent, and
not replicating. Other studies in the *Journal of the American Medical
Association, Cancer Research Institute, Lancet,* and the *New England
Journal of Medicine* have all validated the anti-carcinogenic properties of progesterone as well. While reviewing published research on
progesterone and breast health I found thirteen studies demonstrating
progesterone's ability to prevent breast cancer and/or breast cell proliferation, seven studies showing that progesterone does not increase
risk of breast cancer and one showing the protective role progesterone
plays in breast tissue. Please take a few moments to review them in
the REFERENCES chapter at the end of the book.

How does progesterone do it? It detoxifies potentially toxic
metabolites (by-products) of estrogen in breast tissue, for one thing,
and in many other ways as well. If you or any one you know has, has
had in the past, or is concerned about breast cancer risk, *What Your
Doctor May Not Tell You About Breast Cancer* by John Lee, MD and
David Zava, PhD is an absolute must read. These guys go into great
detail about all of the hormones related to breast cancer and explain
more fully the amazing role progesterone plays in protecting the
breast than I can here. Progesterone also has been shown to reduce
fibrocystic breast disease and reduces premenstrual breast pain.

Progesterone's Role in Preventing Other Cancers

Estrogen's effect on the cells is proliferative-that is, it causes
them to multiply; in contrast, progesterone keeps this proliferation

in check. Progesterone triggers differentiation of cells, instructing them to die off normally. The balancing of estrogen's proliferative properties with progesterone's differentiation property is very important in the prevention of breast and endometrial (uterine lining) cancer; progesterone protects against ovarian cancer as well.

Progesterone and Bones

Progesterone stimulates bone growth by encouraging production of osteoblasts, your bone-building cells. In the early 1990s, Dr. John Lee's research in his medical practice showed that women using progesterone cream experienced an average of 7-8% increase in bone-mineral density in the first year, 4-5% in the second year, and 3-4% in the third year. In a later chapter, we'll discuss the effects of all the sex hormones on osteoporosis.

Progesterone and Skin

Progesterone can even improve your skin. It helps prevent collagen breakdown by stimulating collagen synthesis and promoting the normal actions of collagen and elastin. One research study examining the effects of progesterone cream applied to the skin of perimenopausal and postmenopausal women, found substantial reductions in both number and depth of wrinkles, along with very significant improvement in skin firmness. The data showed a twenty-nine percent reduction in wrinkle counts and depth in the eye area (crow's feet), nine percent decrease in nasolabial wrinkle depth and twenty-three percent skin firmness. Researchers concluded that progesterone is an effective anti-aging cream and can help increase elasticity and firmness in the skin of pre-menopausal and postmenopausal women. I love it when research like this comes out.

Progesterone and Muscles and Connective Tissue

Progesterone affects the function of mitochondria, the powerhouses of energy production in the cells. It also relaxes smooth muscle and reduces spasms. Since progesterone receptors are widely present in submucosal tissue, such as what lines the lungs, sufficient amounts are important for widening the bronchi and regulating mucus. There are even some anecdotal reports of the use of progesterone helping with fibromyalgia.

Progesterone stimulates the injury-healing process in connective tissue by encouraging fibroblast (tissue-building cell) proliferation and thereby soft tissue growth. Studies have also shown progesterone to have an anti-inflammatory effect.

Progesterone's Role in Heart Health

There's even more good news. Progesterone protects you from heart disease by dilating coronary arteries, protecting against atherosclerosis, reducing triglycerides, improving vascular tone, inhibiting blood clotting, increasing HDL (the protective "good" cholesterol) and improving electrical conductions of the heart. Those of you concerned about cholesterol and blood pressure will be happy to hear that progesterone has no negative effect on the lipid profile (your cholesterol and triglycerides) or on C-reactive protein. C-reactive protein is a cardiovascular disease risk factor that results from inflammation.

Progesterone's Role in Stress Tolerance and Sleep

Progesterone increases stress tolerance in several ways. First, it blocks cortisol (the stress hormone) at cortisol receptor sites, and transdermal progesterone cream has been shown to reduce nighttime cortisol levels and to promote normal sleep patterns. These roles are essential if we produce excess cortisol from chronic stress. On the other hand, progesterone serves as the precursor, or raw material, for cortisol production. We do need normal amounts of cortisol, so under stress the body will divert progesterone to cortisol production and control, which can certainly leave us progesterone deficient. Since lack of sleep stimulates cortisol production, better sleep alleviates stress. Second, progesterone fits into the same receptor sites in the brain as valium, morphine, and barbiturates, without addictive effects, which is why progesterone is calming and relaxing and helps with anxiety, irritability, and mood swings. Progesterone activates receptor sites for Gamma Aminobutyric Acid (GABA), a neurotransmitter promoting a calm emotional state.

Progesterone's Role in the Brain/Nervous System

Recent research suggests that progesterone's role in the brain and nervous system is likely a significant one. The brain, spinal cord, and peripheral nerves all actually synthesize small amounts of progesterone from pregnenolone, the grandmother hormone from which all of the other steroid hormones are derived. The brain, in fact, maintains the highest concentration of progesterone of any organ in the body. This is due to its essential role in nerve health and function. If the brain needs high amounts of progesterone, I certainly want mine to have all it needs.

Mouse and rat studies have shown progesterone to be neuroprotective, reducing inflammation and edema after brain injury and promoting formation of myelin sheaths in the brain. This and other research suggests that progesterone may help repair neurological damage as well as treat neurodegenerative diseases and preserve cognitive function that normally declines with age. Other research has shown that patients with Traumatic Brain Injuries on intravenous progesterone were more likely to survive and had better outcomes.

Progesterone's Interactions with Other Hormones

As I mentioned before, progesterone is a balancer of some hormones, particularly estrogen, and is a precursor of other hormones. Since it is metabolized into other hormones like corticosteroids and testosterone, progesterone affects all steroids. We have already talked about progesterone's role as a cortisol blocker, meaning that we need adequate progesterone to oppose cortisol. For people with very low cortisol, it is very important to have progesterone as the precursor to synthesize cortisol. Progesterone is also necessary for thyroid hormone utilization, playing an integral role in the conversion of the thyroid hormone T4 into the much more active thyroid hormone T3 and helping transport thyroid hormone molecules. And estrogen dominance hinders thyroid function because estrogen, especially when taken orally, increases Thyroid Binding Globulin; Thyroid Binding Globulin binds with thyroid hormone just as SHBG binds with estrogen and testosterone and its metabolites, making less thyroid hormone available to the body. Patients with normal thyroid hormone production while estrogen dominant can, therefore, experience functional hypothyroidism, meaning that they have symptoms of hypothyroidism while their thyroid lab results are normal. Low thyroid function, of course, slows metabolism, encouraging weight gain and sapping energy.

More About:

Other Hormones Affected by Progesterone

Corticosteroids (Cortisol): are produced in the adrenal cortex. Corticosteroids play many physiological roles in the body, including in stress response, immune response, regulation of inflammation, carbohydrate metabolism, protein catabolism, blood electrolyte balance, and behavior. Progesterone is required for cortisol synthesis and may help offset elevated cortisol levels.

Thyroxine (T4): T4 is one of the two major hormones secreted by the thyroid gland. Thyroxine's principal function is to stimulate the consumption of oxygen and thus facilitate metabolism in all cells and tissues in the body.

Triiodothyronine (T3): T3 is a thyroid hormone similar to thyroxine but with one less iodine atom per molecule and produced in smaller quantities; it exerts the same biological effects as thyroxine but is more potent and only lasts for a short time in the body.

*Progesterone and progesterone balance with estrogen is necessary for thyroid hormone utilization.

Dihydrotestosterone (DHT): *DHT is a derivative of testosterone produced in various tissues (such as the skin and prostate) that has androgenic activity and anabolic properties. Elevated DHT may cause excess androgen symptoms such as facial hair or acne. Progesterone inhibits the enzyme (5-alpha-reductase) that converts testosterone to DHT.*

Estrogen Deficiency

We're all pretty familiar with common symptoms of estrogen deficiency like hot flashes, night sweats, and insomnia. Because estrogen has a vasodilatory effect (causes blood vessels to dilate), fluctuations in estrogen levels can trigger headaches. The rapid dilation and constriction caused by these fluctuations can also cause hot flashes, night sweats, and heart palpitations. Estrogen deficiency often causes dry skin, dry eyes, and hair loss. Because estrogen helps with carbohydrate metabolism, when estrogen levels drop, women often crave carbohydrates and gain weight. Estrogen deficiency can cause vaginal walls to thin and dry, which can, in turn, cause painful intercourse. It can also increase susceptibility to urinary tract infections and lead to incontinence. And because estrogen regulates the menstrual cycle, it is a drop in estrogen that causes women to stop having periods. As estrogen levels begin to decline or fluctuate, a woman may skip periods, or her periods may become lighter and farther apart.

Estrogen deficiency can also cause many mental and emotional symptoms such as anxiety, depression, loss of motivation, and weepiness. Estrogen-deficient women frequently struggle with foggy thinking, poor verbal recall, and general forgetfulness. Estrogen deficiency increases inflammatory substances in our bodies which affect our brain, bones and cardiovascular health. In short, there's just really nothing good about estrogen deficiency.

Estrogen Deficiency

General Physical Symptoms or Related Conditions:
- *Vasomotor symptoms: hot flashes/night sweats*
- *Headaches*
- *Inflammation*
- *Insomnia or sleep disturbances*
- *Poor memory/concentration or forgetfulness*
- *Hair loss*
- *Dry skin/eyes/hair*
- *Thinning /aging skin and wrinkles*
- *Bone loss*
- *Insulin resistance*
- *Increased cholesterol*
- *Poor carbohydrate metabolism/weight gain*
- *Heart palpitations*
- *Oily skin /acne*
- *Insulin resistance*

Gynecological Symptoms or Related Conditions:
- *Lighter/non-existent periods*
- *Vaginal dryness*
- *Urinary tract infections*
- *Incontinence*

Emotional Symptoms or Related Conditions:
- *Depression*
- *Weepiness*
- *Anxiety*
- *Carbohydrate cravings*
- *Low libido*

What Estrogen Does For You

Estrogen has four hundred crucial functions in the body according to a very comprehensive list compiled by Dr. Pam Smith in her book, *HRT: The Answers*. Estrogen is made by the ovaries as you know. The ovaries make 60% of our estrogen while the other 40% comes from other sources, including the adrenal glands. The body converts androgens such as DHEA, testosterone, and androstenedione made by the adrenals or ovaries into estrogen. We women make approximately 0.01 to 0.03 mg of estradiol (one of the three primary estrogens women make) daily. It is one highly potent hormone.

It's been said that estrogen can be both an angel of light and an angel of death, and it's true. Though we tend to think of estrogen as a dangerous, cancer-causing hormone and though it's true that too much estrogen can cause cancer, too little estrogen can also cause serious problems and some very serious symptoms! No wonder; there are estrogen receptors everywhere in your body. What you really need is just the right amount. As is so often the case, balance is the key. You need just the right amounts, and you need your estrogen and progesterone to balance each other. Most estrogens (there are three primary estrogens) are proliferatory, which causes cells to multiply, notably the breast tissue and other hormone-sensitive tissue. This growth inducing property becomes a problem when unchecked by progesterone. Another innate protective mechanism God gave is metabolism. Estrogen is supposed to be utilized, cleared away in a few hours, and then deactivated promptly. This is referred to as estrogen metabolism, which is performed in part by the liver. The liver requires enzymes, a good supply of nutrients and sulfated amino acids such as cysteine, glutathionine, and methionine. Toxins, rancid fats, stress, and viruses hinder estrogen metabolism.

Though we normally talk about estrogen as one single hormone, our bodies actually produce at least three estrogens: estradiol, estrone, and estriol. Estradiol and estrone are both strong, aggressive, proliferative estrogens, while estriol is believed to be less aggressive. For most of our discussion, we'll lump the three estrogens together and simply refer to estrogen, unless we want to talk about one estrogen in particular.

More About:

The Three Primary Estrogens:

Estradiol - is the strongest estrogen. It is 12 times stronger than estrone and 80 times stronger than estriol. Estradiol is mostly made by the ovaries and is the most abundant estrogen produced premenopausally.

Estrone - is the main hormone produced post-menopausally. High levels of estrone are considered a risk factor for breast and uterine cancer. Estrone can be converted to estradiol and vice versa. Estrone can be made in the fat cells and the adrenal glands.

Estriol - is a non-stimulating estrogen to the breast and uterine tissue. It plays protective roles in the body.

Of course, estrogen plays a big role in every woman's life by regulating her menstrual cycle. Even before the cycles begin, it is estrogen that causes us to develop breasts and our feminine hips and thighs in puberty. It prepares the blood lining and stimulates breast tissue each month in preparation for possible pregnancy. Estrogen causes the egg to mature and creates the follicle where the egg matures. It ensures that the vaginal tissue, vulva, and cervix are developed and moisturized. Since estrogen plays a role in temperature regulation, as menopause approaches, estrogen deficiency and/ or rapid fluctuations in estrogen levels can trigger symptoms like hot flashes and night sweats, so adequate estrogen prevents many miseries associated with menopause.

Estrogen's Effects on the Urogenital Region

Estrogen increases vaginal elasticity and promotes vascularity (thickens blood vessels) of the urogenital region. This increased vascularity increases vaginal discharge, relieving vaginal dryness and therefore preventing painful intercourse. Greater vascularity also helps prevent urogenital atrophy, atrophic vaginitis, urinary tract infections, dysuria (painful or difficult urination), and urinary urgency. A 1993 study published in the *New England Journal of Medicine* showed that estrogens, estriol in particular, helps prevent urinary tract infections, and several other studies have reached the same conclusion.

More About:

Atrophic Vaginitis

Atrophic vaginitis: inflammation of the vaginal mucosa due to thinning and decreased lubrication of the vaginal walls. This condition is typically caused by estrogen deficiency. Common symptoms include vaginal soreness, vaginal itching, pain with intercourse, and possible bleeding after intercourse. Treatment includes intra-vaginal estrogen cream or raising systemic levels of estrogen.

Estrogen's Effects on the Heart

Estrogen protects your heart by managing blood pressure (by acting as a calcium channel blocker and relaxing the lining of the blood vessels), raising HDL (good cholesterol), lowering LDL (bad cholesterol), lowering triglycerides, lowering fibrinogen (associated with clotting), and dilating blood vessels to improve blood flow. Estrogen plays an important role in maintaining elasticity of the arteries and decreases the accumulation of plaque. It also has antioxidant properties and has been shown to decrease other risk factors now associated with heart disease: lipoprotein (a) and homocysteine. According to Dr. Sinatra in his book, *Heart Sense for Women,* estrogen decreases the over all risk of heart disease in women 40 to 50 percent.

Many women go through their thirties and forties with normal levels of cholesterol and normal blood pressure. Then, with the onset of menopause, if their estrogen drops to deficiency range, up goes their cholesterol level or their blood pressure. Common sense tells us you don't use estrogen to lower cholesterol or address hypertension if you don't have low estrogen levels. You must have appropriate treatment per your doctor.

Estrogen's Effects on Bones

We've all heard that estrogen protects against osteoporosis, but how? It does so by subduing osteoclasts (cells that break down old bone tissue), thereby slowing bone resorption. Bone resorption is a normal bone cell activity. In very general terms it is the process of resorbing or removing old cells. The bottom line is that if estrogen levels drop too low, osteoclasts remove the old bone faster than your body can replace it. Excessive osteoclast activity also occurs during the time just before and during the cessation of menstrual cycles. This is due to the reduction of estrogen production, which in turn leads to menopause. Moreover, estrogen controls the absorption of calcium into the bone and stimulates production of calcitonin-the hormone that protects bone. (Please see Chapter 7 for a detailed discussion of bone building and osteoporosis.)

Estrogen's Effects on the Brain

According to Dr. Frederick Naftolin who has served as professor and chairman of Yale Medical School's Department of Obstetrics and Gynecology, clinical chief of the Ob/Gyn Department at Yale-New Haven Hospital and a leading officer of the North American Menopause Society, "There is not a cell in the brain that is not directly or indirectly sensitive to estrogen." Estrogen supports brain function in many important ways, especially in memory and verbal memory, visual-spatial memory, perception, speech and language skills, concentration, problem solving, higher-order intellectual functioning, attention span, and the processing of incoming information. Name recall is improved in women taking estrogen. Estrogen protects your brain and prevents memory disorders. It delays and decreases the risk of developing Alzheimer's disease. In fact, research has shown that women taking estrogen are only half as likely to develop Alzheimer's compared to those not taking it. Conversely, research on HRT shows it does not demonstrate this protection. One way estrogen accomplishes all these great things is by increasing the levels of neurotransmitters like acetylcholine, serotonin, dopamine, epinephrine, and norepinephrine. Normal levels of these neurotransmitters improve alertness, reaction time, verbal ability, and mood. Low serotonin levels trigger depression and cravings for carbohydrates.

More About:

Neurotransmitters

Neurotransmitters are chemicals required for proper brain and body function; without them, our nervous system would fail and we would lose the ability to think, feel, act, and function in a way that keeps our bodies healthy and our mind alive. When neurotransmitters are not functioning properly we can experience all types of symptoms and health problems.

Listed below are a few neurotransmitters that are directly affected by estrogen.

Serotonin: Constricts blood vessels at injury sites, affects emotional states, sense of well-being, is involved in sleep, depression, memory, and other neurological processes.

Dopamine: Acts within the brain to help regulate movement, brain function, coordination and emotion, is a precursor of epinephrine; its depletion may cause Parkinson's disease.

Epinephrine: Produced by the adrenal gland that stimulates muscle tissue and raises blood pressure; also called adrenaline. Optimal levels are very important for memory, focus and concentration.

Norepinephrine: Secreted by the adrenal gland and similar to epinephrine, it increases blood pressure, blood flow to the brain, and rate and depth of breathing. It raises the level of blood sugar, confidence, and motivation.

Estrogen also encourages the transport of glucose and oxygen across the blood-brain barrier. Since glucose is what fuels your brain, it is essential to have adequate amounts supplied to the brain.

Estrogen's Role in Sleep

Estrogen reduces the amount of time it takes to get to sleep and increases the REM or deep sleep, thereby greatly improving the quality of our sleep. For many menopausal women suffering from insomnia, realizing this amazing role of estrogen can be life changing.

Estrogen's Role in Metabolism and Weight

Estradiol in the proper amount helps prevent weight gain by improving carbohydrate metabolism while increasing sensitivity of muscle and fat tissue to insulin. Estrogen stimulates the production of lipoprotein lipase, an enzyme that breaks down fat (including cholesterol). In regard to weight, insulin encourages fat storage and estrogen helps lower insulin. On the other hand, excess estrogen actually impairs glucose tolerance. Once again, balance is key.

New research has found that women low in estrogen have higher levels of the stress hormone cortisol, thus more abdominal weight gain. On July 15, 2005, Oregon Health & Science University researchers unveiled research results that help explain why middle-aged women develop central body fat. "These findings also suggest that estrogen replacement therapy protects women from developing high cortisol levels and increased abdominal fat," said Jonathan Purnell, M.D., an associate professor of medicine (endocrinology, diabetes and clinical nutrition) in the OHSU School of Medicine and a researcher in OHSU's Center for the Study of Weight Regulation and Associated Disorders. Purnell continued, "We believe that by preventing this rise in cortisol we can possibly delay or prevent weight issues and the many weight-associated disorders in some of these women." To further confirm the relationship between estrogen replacement and cortisol levels, researchers treated seven postmenopausal women not already undergoing HRT with estrogen. (This study used a synthetic form of estrogen.) After one month of therapy, these women, who all previously had heightened cortisol levels, had cortisol levels similar to those typical of premenopausal women.

Another potential way estrogen affects weight is in regard to ghrelin. Ghrelin is a hormone that makes you hungrier, more focused on food and willing to eat more. Transdermal estradiol has been shown to decrease ghrelin, increase satiety and decrease food intake. Transdermal estradiol has been shown to help with weight and insulin resistance. Ladies please, this preliminary research is not reason enough to run out and ask your doctor for a prescription. Lab work documenting low or low-normal estrogen levels are the only real grounds for replacing estrogen.

Estrogen's Effects on Skin, Eyes and Mouth

In addition to promoting eye and oral health, estrogen plays an enormous role in the health of your skin. It increases the moisture content of skin by pulling water into cells and increases production of type II collagen and hyaluronic acid-major components of skin involved in tissue repair.

More About:

Collagen

Collagen is the main protein of connective tissue. Tough bundles of collagen called collagen fibers give cells structure from the outside, but collagen is also found inside certain cells. Collagen is the main component of fascia, cartilage, ligaments, tendons, bone, and teeth. Along with soft keratin, it is responsible for skin strength and elasticity, and its degradation leads to wrinkles that accompany aging. It also strengthens blood vessels and plays a role in tissue development. It is present in the cornea and lens of the eye as well.

Estrogen also maintains skin thickness, reduces pore size and wrinkle depth, and is useful to speed wound healing. As you can see, estrogen is necessary to your skin's health and very helpful in slowing the aging process. The estrogen estriol is proving exceptionally helpful in this regard. Estrogen has also been shown to reduce risk of cataracts and macular degeneration, improve visual function, prevent intraocular pressure and improve amount/quality of eye lubrication. In addition, it helps prevent tooth loss.

Estrogen's Effect on Nutrients

Estrogen helps maintain potassium levels and helps with absorption of calcium, magnesium and zinc.

Estriol

As I mentioned, there are three primary estrogens that women's bodies produce: estradiol (also referred to as E2), estrone (also referred to as E1) and Estriol (also referred to as E3). Estriol is the most widely prescribed estrogen in Europe. Unfortunately, most American doctors don't even know about it. Estriol is different from the other two estrogens. Because estriol appears to be a less aggressive proliferatory agent than estradiol and estrone, it, therefore, appears less likely to cause cancer. Women with a history of breast cancer that have been told not to use estradiol often turn to estriol for its beneficial and symptom relieving properties. Many BHRT specialists prescribe Biest, which is a combination of estriol and estradiol. It provides a small amount of the powerful estradiol with the additional benefits of estriol. Estrone is no longer used in BHRT. This is because giving estradiol will increase estrone adequately. Excess estrone can form carcinogenic metabolites.

Even estriol used alone (without the other estrogens) can address many estrogen-deficiency symptoms. A summary of the research conducted on estriol includes the following: it relieves hot flashes and reduces vaginal dryness, painful intercourse, vaginal atrophy, dysuria (pain or difficulty in urinating), and urinary urgency. It also helps prevent urinary tract infections, according to a 1993 *New England Journal of Medicine* study among others. Estriol has also been shown to increases bone mass 1-5% over twelve months of use and to reduce the excretion of calcium. Other studies have shown that estriol lowers both total cholesterol and LDL (bad cholesterol) while raising HDL (good cholesterol). It also lowers triglycerides and doesn't increase blood clotting. Surprisingly, estriol may even protect against breast and uterine cancer. When estriol was given to women with metastatic breast cancer in the 1970s, 37% saw remission or arrest of lesions. One researcher found that estriol inhibited formation of radiation- and carcinogen-induced rat mammary carcinomas by 80%. And some research indicates that estriol deficiencies may be associated with breast cancer.

Newer research also seemed to document Estriol's ability to protect against breast cancer. For example, an unpublished paper reported on 15,000 women followed for thirty-five to forty years. They found that breast cancer risk was reduced 58 percent in women with the highest levels of estriol compared to the lowest levels. Another study published in the *International Journal of Cancer* in 2004 found that women using estriol cream or pills in their HRT did not have an increased risk of breast cancer at all.

Estriol is both pro-estrogenic and anti-estrogenic, and this may explain why estriol may play a protective role in regard to breast cancer. When estriol is given with the more aggressive estradiol as in Biest, the estradiol stimulation to cells is decreased. When taken alone, estriol is more stimulatory in its actions. Interestingly, there are two types of estrogen receptors in the breast tissue: estrogen receptor alpha and estrogen receptor beta. When an estrogen binds to the estrogen receptor alpha there is promotion of cell proliferation which can lead to breast cancer if left uncontrolled by the body (and progesterone). Conversely, the binding of estrogen to estrogen receptor beta inhibits cell proliferation and may possibly prevent breast cancer development. As you may have suspected, estradiol and estrone bind to estrogen receptor alpha while estriol binds to estrogen receptor beta.

In regard to the skin, a study on estriol reported in the *International Journal of Dermatology* in 1995 found that after seven to ten weeks of treatment with topical estriol 100% of subjects reported flattening of acne scars, and 77% reported pore shrinkage. This is good news for women of all ages, and it does have wonderful effects on aging skin. Topical estriol has been shown to reverse wrinkling, increase skin moisture, improve the skin's blood supply, and increase elasticity and firmness while reducing pore size and wrinkle depth. It boosts levels of type II collagen, which speeds healing, and hyaluronic acid, which keeps skin plump and helps it retain moisture. It kind of makes you want to bathe in the stuff, doesn't it?

Unfortunately, at the time of this writing, a prominent pharmaceutical company is trying to get the FDA to keep you from having access to estriol, even by prescription.

More About:

Estriol – Summary of Research

- *Controls menopausal symptoms of hot flashes, insonnia and vaginal dryness*
- *Helps maintain good bacteria in gut*
- *Has positive effects on the vaginal lining*
- *Increases HDL (good cholesterol) and lowers LDL (bad cholesterol)*
- *Restores proper pH of vagina which may help prevent urinary tract infections*
- *Has been used to treat breast cancer; studies indicate it may prevent breast cancer*

A Special Note to Women Who Have Had a Hysterectomy Taking Estrogen Only Therapy (ERT) Without Progesterone

Traditional medical training instructs physicians to prescribe estrogen-only therapy for women who have had their ovaries removed from having had a hysterectomy. It may be an estrogen patch, which is bioidentical, or an oral synthetic or animal-derived form of estrogen. Here is the problem: the standard of care is that a woman without a uterus does not need a progestin (synthetic progesterone) to protect her from increased risk of endometrial cancer from the estrogen. This is true; women don't need the synthetic progesterone and its side effects, but what about the crucial role progesterone plays in preventing breast cancer, protecting the heart and skin, building bone, etc., as we have reviewed earlier? Because there is a progesterone receptor in every cell of a women's body, we need progesterone for it's many other vital roles. These women are entitled to the many amazing roles progesterone plays in health too

Testosterone Deficiency

It's not hard to figure out the symptoms of testosterone deficiency in women. Given testosterone's reputation, it's not surprising that testosterone deficiency affects libido and can even cause female sexual arousal disorder (FSAD) and sexual dysfunction. It can also cause vaginal dryness and incontinence. Since testosterone is an anabolic (tissue building) steroid, testosterone deficiency can lead to muscular atrophy, bone loss, and thinning of skin. Testosterone deficiency can also cause fatigue, aches and pains, arthritic pain in particular, and myofascial pain (pain in the fascia, which is the soft tissue component of the connective tissue). Myofascial pain is associated with and caused by "trigger points" (sensitive and painful areas between the muscles and fascia), fibromyalgic symptoms, and a much lower tolerance for pain in general. Low levels of testosterone are also associated with depression and poor memory. So women really need testosterone, and we don't want to be deficient. On the other hand, you really don't want to have too much testosterone either.

Testosterone Deficiency Symptoms

General Physical Symptoms or Related Conditions:
- *Vasomotor symptoms: hot flashes/night sweats*
- *Aches and pains*
- *Fatigue*
- *Insomnia*
- *Poor memory*
- *Thinning skin*
- *Loss of muscle tone*
- *Bone loss*

- *Heart palpitations*

Gynecological Symptoms or Related Conditions:
- *Loss or thinning of pubic hair*
- *Vaginal dryness*
- *Incontinence*
- *Lichen sclerosus*
- *Loss of libido*
- *Impaired sexual function or female sexual arousal disorder*

Emotional Symptoms or Related Conditions:
- *Depression*
- *Lack of motivation*
- *Low self-esteem*
- *Hypersensitive*
- *Anxiety*

What Testosterone Does for You

Women make around 0.3 mg of testosterone daily, which is about ten times more than estrogen. The ovaries make approximately 60% of the total testosterone. The rest comes from DHEA contribution, which is made by the adrenal glands.

Testosterone is responsible for building structural tissue like bone, skin, and muscle, so women do require and produce testosterone. Testosterone maintains lean body mass, strength, and stamina; it helps increase muscle bulk and tone. Because testosterone increases support of the levator ani, a muscle that supports the abdomen and urogenital region and sphincter muscles, testosterone-deficient women sometimes leak urine. Testosterone is important to skeletal health too, aiding in the formation of strong bones and thereby reducing fractures. It does so by increasing bone mineral density.

Like other steroid hormones, testosterone plays an important role in cardiovascular health. In both men and women, the heart contains the largest concentration of testosterone receptors of the whole body, demonstrating the importance of adequate levels of testosterone for the heart. Testosterone also improves blood flow to the heart.

This hormone protects the brain too, supporting the structural integrity of the brain and assisting in the synthesis of the neurotransmitters dopamine, epinephrine, norepinephrine, and acetylcholine. Adequate levels of these neurotransmitters encourage a sense of well-being and improve mood, help combat depression, increases energy, self-esteem, and memory. Interestingly, the brain requires estrogen for testosterone to attach to brain receptors.

Other vital roles testosterone plays are creating energy and regulating the immune system. Testosterone affects hair growth. Many women with testosterone deficiency have thinning scalp hair or loss of pubic hair. They often state that they don't have to shave their legs very often anymore and have less hair on their arms.

More About:

Testosterone – A Summary of Research

- *May decrease nearly 50% by mid-forties*
- *Reduces women's fear response*
- *Used to treat depression*
- *Improves sexual response*
- *Builds bone*
- *Low levels associated with heart disease including hardening of the arteries*
- *May be protective against breast cancer*
- *May be helpful and preventive in treating diabetes*
- *Oral contraceptives lower testosterone*
- *Women may lose 70% of testosterone with removal of ovaries*
- *No virilizing or adverse events seen with low dosing*

Excessive Testosterone

The ovaries produce 60% of the testosterone in a woman's body, but an ovarian cyst can cause the ovaries to produce excess testosterone. More often, insulin resistance causes testosterone excess in women because excess insulin stimulates the ovaries to produce more androgens (hormones with masculinizing effects), including testosterone and increases DHEA. Excess testosterone can cause mid-cycle pain, oily skin, acne, and facial hair. Loss of scalp hair, specifically male-pattern type baldness in women, is another symptom, although this can also be due to low levels of estrogen or progesterone. (As mentioned earlier, testosterone affects hair growth therefore low testosterone can also trigger hair loss.) Higher than normal levels of testosterone can cause breast pain and raise the risk of breast cancer. Not surprisingly, excess androgens can also make a woman overly aggressive and irritable.

Symptoms of Excess Testosterone

• *Acne/oily skin*
• *Facial hair*
• *Thinning scalp hair*
• *Excess body hair*
• *Mid-cycle pain (at ovulation)*
• *Pain in nipples*
• *Ovarian cysts*
• *Hypoglycemia or insulin resistance*
• *Elevated triglycerides*
• *Aggression, irritability*

Importance of Hormone Balance

Even if you have no symptoms of hormone imbalance or are willing to put up with unpleasant symptoms, hormone imbalances can cause or be associated with serious conditions like obesity, hypothyroidism, chronic fatigue, metabolic syndrome, polycystic ovarian syndrome, luteal phase insufficiency (a common cause of infertility), uterine fibroids, depression, mood disorders, premenstrual dysphoric disorder, memory disorders, seizure disorders, insomnia, fatigue, migraines, asthma, connective tissue diseases, skin disorders, hirsutism (excess facial hair in women), and bone loss. You can see how serious hormone problems can be. In the next chapter, we'll look at different ways to address hormone imbalances and deficiencies.

Chapter 4

THE HORMONE MAKEOVER

Seven Steps in the Hormone Makeover

1. Find a BHRT physician.
2. Get prepared to work with a BHRT physician.
3. Test your hormones.
4. Correct imbalances with bioidentical hormones, appropriate supplements, and dietary or lifestyle changes.
5. Manage imbalances of related hormones: adrenals, insulin and thyroid.
6. Address specific conditions such as PMS, bone loss or breast cysts with indicated therapies.
7. Love yourself enough to invest in you.

The remainder of this book will cover each of these steps one by one in great detail. Use them as a resource before and during the course of your hormone makeover process.

Throughout this book, we've seen how hormone imbalances profoundly affect us physically, mentally, emotionally, and even spiritually. Balancing your hormones should alleviate menstrual symptoms as well as the problems of perimenopause and menopause. Once your hormones are balanced, you should be able to sleep better and manage your weight more easily. You will feel emotionally stable and get back to feeling like yourself again. You might even experience greater intimacy with God once you stop needing to repent so often for things you said or did when your hormones were raging. You'll have the joy of being able to serve God without the hindrances of hormonal headaches, heavy-to-the-point-of-flooding menstrual flow, or hormonally induced depression. And in the long run, balanced hormones may help you avoid diseases or conditions connected with hormone deficiencies. You'll have a better chance of enjoying the long, rich life God has ordained for you, and you will decrease your risk of developing age-related diseases associated with hormone imbalances, like osteoporosis and cardiovascular disease. So let's get down to the nitty-gritty of implementing your hormone makeover.

STEP ONE: FIND A BHRT PHYSICIAN

Don't Go It Alone

The first thing you need to consider from the outset is that it's extremely difficult, and in most cases impossible, to go it alone. Sure, you can study and learn a lot on your own, but you still need hormone testing and monitoring, for which you really need the help of a highly trained BHRT health-care practitioner. So, how do you find a good one? The good news is that there are many more health care providers out there writing prescriptions for BHRT now than there used to be. It's a great blessing, but it's a little tricky because a lot of them aren't really experts in BHRT. Prescribing BHRT can be quite complicated, and many practitioners prescribing it haven't had the in-depth training they need. It's not a one-dose-fits-all therapy; it truly has to be customized to each patient, which means that it takes a fair amount of time. In my experience, an initial BHRT consultation takes about an hour because the practitioner needs to go over a woman's medical history and hormone-related symptoms and answer all her questions. Every woman has a different story and deserves to be heard; we all need an opportunity to voice our personal concerns. You just can't do all that in fifteen minutes, and most medical practices just aren't set up to give each patient an hour. So how do you find someone with adequate training who is willing to spend the necessary time to tailor BHRT to your needs?

There are several ways to go about finding a good BHRT practitioner. You can contact hormone-testing labs, such as ZRT, Aeron LifeCycles, or Labrix, through their web sites and ask for names of the health-care providers in your area who are ordering these special hormone tests. Or you can call your local compounding pharmacist. (Compounding pharmacies prepare customized doses of the precise hormones in the specific amounts you need.) Many compounding pharmacists have received training in BHRT, and they can tell you which medical offices are sending them prescriptions for compounded bioidentical hormones. In fact, many compounding pharmacists trained in BHRT do hormone consultations for local physicians. Health food stores can also be a valuable resource. People who work there can often point you to local BHRT experts. I hardly need mention your friends as possible referral sources. Women who have found relief from hormone woes are seldom reticent to mention it to their friends. You probably know several women who talk on and on about how much better they feel since they started seeing so-and-so about their hormones.

Since some areas don't have any BHRT practitioners, you may have to drive farther than you'd like, but it's worth it. And the good news is that achieving hormone balance doesn't usually require lots of trips to the BHRT professional. As a general rule, you should expect to make at least two initial visits and another visit three to six months later. After that, six month to yearly visits usually suffice. Of course, the schedule can vary, depending on your situation and the practitioner. Some practitioners will conduct minor dosing adjustments by phone.

One more important note: don't overlook nurse practitioners and physicians' assistants in your search for a BHRT practitioner. The reason I keep using terms like "health-care practitioner" and "health-care provider" instead of "doctor" is that many BHRT practitioners are nurse practitioners (NP) and physicians' assistants (PA) rather than doctors, and many of them are highly skilled in BHRT. In most states they can treat patients just like MDs. It often works out that you can have your BHRT consultations with an NP or a PA in the same office where you receive your OB/GYN care.

When you find someone you might want to provide your BHRT care, screen the practitioner by talking to the administrative staff in the office. Ask if he or she orders hormone testing, whether he or she uses nutritional supplements, how long the practitioner has been prescribing BHRT, and how many patients he or she has worked with.

If you cannot find an experienced BHRT physician in your area you are welcome to make an appointment with us at Signature Wellness in Charlotte, NC. For additional support I invite you to visit my web site for an array of resources to help you through your hormone makeover process. I am most excited about our live and archived web shows and hormone balancing classes. This is a great place for women to be introduced to BHRT, get in-depth education on hormones and how to get them back into balance, ask specific questions and hear feedback from other women. The information, resources and updates on BHRT are there to help you. Take full advantage of every opportunity. Very soon, my staff and I will be able to help your doctor in your area learn the mechanics of how to give you a hormone makeover.

Resources:

www.donnawhitehormonemakeover.com
www.signaturewellness.org
http://hormonemakeover.blogspot.com

STEP 2: GET PREPARED TO WORK WITH YOUR BHRT PHYSICIAN

Once you're satisfied that you've found a good BHRT practitioner, set up an appointment and make sure you're prepared ahead of time so you can make the most of your visit. First, be ready to discuss your medical history or write it on the intake forms. Pertinent information includes dates of past surgeries, past illnesses, and answers to any of the myriad questions those forms usually list. Be sure you know your family medical history, especially regarding hormone-related cancers. Take along a written list of medications as well as herbs and supplements you're taking, both prescription and OTC. Be sure to include dosages. I would recommend that you get copies of any recent lab test results (within the last year) and take them with you. Be sure to let the practitioner know that you have them. These can provide valuable information and possibly save you money by avoiding unnecessary testing. By the way, always ask for and keep copies of all lab test results and keep them in a file. That way you won't have to request them later if you move or the practice closes or whatever. Some doctors' offices now charge a fee to copy your medical records, an expense you might be able to avoid if you always ask for lab test results immediately. And having your own copies can help you manage your own case by tracking changes in your cholesterol, thyroid hormones, etc.

Your menstrual history will be important to discuss, so know the length of your cycles and periods. If you haven't been keeping track, you can start now. (There's a chart on my web site you can copy: www.donnawhitehormonemakeover.com. Some of our patients have downloaded applications on their phones that keep track of their cycles.) Think about any symptoms or problems related to your periods. For example, if you always get a headache the day before you start your period, be sure to mention it.

Be ready to list and discuss any medical treatments you have tried and how you responded to them. I would also suggest that you gather (and possibly put into writing) your thoughts about three things: 1) your symptoms if you have more than a very few, 2) your questions, and 3) your goals. For instance, you may be most concerned about immediate symptoms like hot flashes, or you may be more concerned with preventing bone loss. Your BHRT provider needs to focus first on what's most important to you.

You may want to keep all this information and your medical records in a notebook so you can prepare for all future appointments with a minimum of effort. After all, no one else can manage your health as well as you. Even if you have a highly skilled BHRT provider, it's still up to you to keep up with everything. Be sure to make a place in your notebook to keep track of the dosages of hormones and supplements you're taking and how you respond. For example, if a certain dosage of some hormone makes you sleepy if you take it in the morning or if a certain amount of some supplement tends to keep you awake at night, make a note of it for future reference. All this information will enable your provider to work out a better treatment protocol for you.

Even if you have found a wonderful BHRT physician you can benefit greatly and experience an optimal outcome by joining me and other women on our web show.
(See www.donnawhitehormonemakeover.com)

Only My Opinion

As BHRT has grown more popular, the medical profession has devised many different approaches to administering it. Like all BHRT practitioners, I have my own approach based on years of experience in preparing treatment protocols for the doctors I've worked with. What I'm sharing with you is what I have seen work. What other practitioners prescribe may be very effective, but I can only share the highly effective protocols the medical doctors I have worked with over the past ten years utilize for patients.

Please understand that as I explain how to implement BHRT, I am not attempting to prescribe or recommend anything specific for anyone. I am laying out ideas so that you can take whichever ones you think might apply to you and discuss them with a highly trained BHRT practitioner. Do not try to treat yourself. This book is meant to help you understand a little more about your hormones so that you will know exactly what questions to ask your BHRT practitioner. Since your health care providers can't possibly explain everything to you at your office visits, I hope to fill in the gaps or even lay a foundation of knowledge that can help you achieve optimal results.

STEP 3: TEST YOUR HORMONES

Starting Your Hormone Makeover
Requires Hormone Testing

The third step in the hormone makeover is hormone testing. You have to know your current hormone levels before you start treatment. Besides, there is nothing like seeing the reason for all your symptoms right there in front of you in black and white. So many women have told me they were afraid their test results would come back normal, and they'd know they were crazy or imagining their symptoms. After the initial test, you will need follow-up hormone testing at least four weeks to three months after initiating therapy to ensure that you're getting the right dose. Thereafter, you should be tested yearly or semi-annually. Remember, women respond very differently to hormones, and you only need exactly what you need, neither more nor less.

Of course, to be of any use to you, hormone testing must be accurate. Though blood tests are ideal for testing thyroid hormones, insulin, and blood sugar, the most accurate method of testing sex and adrenal hormones is the saliva test. Blood and urine tests are much less effective for testing these hormones because of the phenomenon we mentioned in Chapter 3; hormones travel through the blood stream in one of two states: bound and free. Hormones traveling through the body eventually pass through the liver, where they bind with a protein coat called SHBG (Sex Hormone Binding Globulin). Actually, 95 to 99% of the hormones in the blood are protein bound. The problem with blood and urine tests of hormone levels is that they can't distinguish between bound and free hormones. In fact, even hormone metabolites, or by-products, are indistinguishable from functional hormones in blood and urine tests, so these tests may indicate that you have abundant levels of hormones when only a fraction of that amount is functional.

What you really need to know from your test is the level of free hormones capable of attaching to the receptor sites in your cells in order to perform their function. Because only free hormones and not bound hormones can pass into the salivary glands, only free hormones end up in your saliva. Therefore, a test of hormone levels in your saliva gives you the information you need, which is the level of "bio-available" hormones—hormones available to your body tissues.

The bottom line is that saliva tests reveal how hormones are working for you where you need them. Saliva hormone testing also more accurately reflects tissue uptake and response of hormones delivered topically (through the skin) in creams, gels, or patches. Blood and urine assays significantly underestimate hormones delivered topically, often resulting in overdosing. Developed in part by world-renowned breast cancer researcher David Zava, Ph.D., saliva testing has been used in scientific research for decades, and it has been shown to be highly accurate; even the World Health Organization has recognized this hormone-testing method, and NASA and the US government use it.

Saliva testing has been a tremendous help to women everywhere and an enormous boon to women whose blood tests show adequate hormone levels but whose symptoms point to hormone deficiencies. If you have heard that there is no scientific validation of saliva testing, that statement simply is not a fact. The references are in the bibliography and on my web site for your convenience. Some BHRT practitioners do use blood tests instead, but the reference ranges (ranges of normal hormone levels) are so broad as to make accurate treatment dosing somewhat of a guess. Again, blood tests do not give tissue levels of hormones; they only give levels found in the blood.

Note: Please use a saliva testing kit ordered by your physician versus an over the counter test kit from a retail store. Those retail kits are typically not comprehensive enough. If your doctor does not offer saliva testing, you can order one from my web site: www.donnawhitehormonemakeover.com.

When You Should Wait Until Later To Do Your Saliva Test

Since knowing your current hormone levels is vital to your hormone makeover, accurate hormone testing is essential. Therefore, your first step will usually be figuring out which tests you need based on your symptoms. Since most of the symptoms we're discussing in this book point to imbalances in sex hormones, adrenal hormones, thyroid hormones, or blood sugar, you'll probably need to test your sex, adrenal, and thyroid hormones. In some cases, you may also need to test your fasting insulin and blood sugar. There are, however, three situations in which hormone testing probably shouldn't be your first step.

1.) If you are currently taking HRT (Combination estrogen/ synthetic progesterone), you should wait to test.

If you're on non-bioidentical HRT, that is, synthetic or animal-derived hormones, hormone testing will be a waste of money, especially if you plan to stop taking them anyway. Tests cannot measure a synthetic hormone level. To get an accurate test, you'd have to stop taking them four weeks before testing. You can certainly do that, but you might get pretty uncomfortable by the time you take your test. As an alternative, if you know you feel better on hormones, you can talk to your BHRT practitioner about just starting you on a low dose of BHRT (see sections below on forms and starting dosages of estrogens and progesterone), so you can hang on until you can test your hormones and review the results with your BHRT provider. This means that you will switch directly from HRT to BHRT at your first visit. Then, after being on BHRT for four to six weeks, you can test. Based on knowledge and experience, the BHRT provider will guess at the proper dose to begin with, but certainly after seeing your test results, he or she can adjust the dose accordingly. If your test results show imbalances of any hormones your practitioner will address these imbalances at that time. This approach can minimize hormonal disruption during the switch from HRT to BHRT.

2.) If you are on ERT (estrogen only), you should wait to test.

You probably also don't want to test your hormones right away if you are on estrogen-only therapy (ERT). Doctors normally pre-scribe ERT for women who have had hysterectomies under the outdated assumption that since you don't have to worry about endo-metrial cancer, you don't need progesterone. (Please see Special Note to Women Who Have Had Hysterectomies with Removal of Ovaries on Estrogen Only Therapy in Chapter 3.) I'll belabor the point I made in that section. You do need progesterone. No matter what anyone has told you, if you're getting supplemental estrogen, you need supplemental progesterone too. A quick look at the list of progesterone's properties and effects in Chapter 3 will convince you. Your BHRT physician will likely suggest you use proges-terone for about four weeks before performing your hormone test. If you are on bioidentical estrogen, preferably transdermal (applied to the skin as a cream, gel, or patch), you can add progesterone, transdermal cream or gel, and then test your hormones in about four to six weeks. Note: If you are on oral estrogen (even bioidentical estradiol), I strongly urge you to consider changing to transdermal application. Oral bioidentical hormones can trigger side effects because they are altered in the digestive tract to form metabolites which can lead to blood clots to mention just one down side. (See the comparison of oral medication versus transdermal treatment given later in this chapter.)

3.) If you are on birth control, you should wait to test.

Also consider delaying hormone testing if you're using synthetic hormonal birth control, such as the pill, the patch, etc. Hormone testing doesn't measure levels of synthetic hormones in your body, so any tests will typically show low levels of estrogen, progesterone, and often even testosterone. Synthetic hormones suppress normal hormone production, and hormone testing will not show how much of each hormone your body is capable of producing. The same holds true if you have an intrauterine device (IUD) or intrauterine system (IUS) that emits synthetic progesterone; obviously, in this case, the only way to get an accurate test is to have it removed. As we've seen, synthetic progesterone doesn't do all the wonderful things that natural progesterone does for you. Neither can synthetic estrogen or testosterone for that matter.

Some birth control pills also contain testosterone receptor blockers, which naturally reduce testosterone. This could be a good thing if your testosterone is too high, of course, but a bad thing if your testosterone is too low. If you choose to continue hormonal birth control, please bear in mind the effects it will have on your hormone levels when you look at your test results. If, on the other hand, you plan to stop taking the pill, stop at the end of the pack and test next cycle on Day 21. If you're using birth control hormones to manage severe PMS or other menstrual problems like cramps or heavy periods, you may be afraid to stop for fear of the return of symptoms. You may want to talk to your health care provider about switching to natural progesterone only (no estrogen for now) and following good nutritional protocols designed to prevent these problems. Then, test on Day 21 of your next cycle. Your test results will show what other steps to take to get relief from these symptoms. There are ways to conquer these problems without having to take hormonal birth control.

Taking a Saliva Test

I suggest a minimum five-panel test that measures estradiol, progesterone, testosterone, DHEA, and morning cortisol; this test automatically includes the ratio of estradiol to progesterone. Beware of BHRT consultation services or providers who only check estradiol and progesterone. Also beware of those who test estradiol, progesterone, and testosterone only. It is essential to check the levels of the adrenal hormones, DHEA and cortisol. True hormone balance cannot be reached without addressing adrenal hormone imbalances.

Since the saliva test must be performed first thing in the morning, you do it yourself at home after obtaining the test kit from your BHRT practitioner. After taking the test, you will mail the specimen to the lab, following the instructions included in the kit. The kit even includes a shipping envelope and postage, so it's easy. The lab will send a report directly to your practitioner in five to seven days after receiving your sample. Be sure to get a copy of these results for your records. One thing you need to be aware of is that some saliva testing labs are considerably more reputable than others. Unfortunately, some labs don't have adequate quality control, and some do not remove contaminants from the samples before testing. Results from these labs may not help you reach your goal of hormone balance. The best labs, of course, remove contaminants and have excellent quality control. I also prefer labs that take your age, menstrual status, symptoms, and use of hormones into account in their lab reports.

Collection Instructions

Women still menstruating will normally collect saliva on Day 19, 20, or 21 of the menstrual cycle. Check with your doctor to be sure when he wants you to test. Non-menstruating women may collect any day. Women having irregular cycles will have to check with the doctor ordering the test.

Test kits come with a requisition form that should be marked by the doctor as to what hormones to check. Again, we typically check a minimum of estradiol, progesterone, testosterone, DHEA, and cortisol. Be sure to read the testing instructions included in the kit the night before your test so you'll be prepared in the morning.

Saliva testing is very easy, and it is great for people who don't like needles. Because you must collect it within the first hour of rising, you will perform the test first thing in the morning before you eat or drink anything or brush your teeth and before using any hormone creams. Allow extra time the morning of your test because sample collection takes about fifteen to thirty minutes. You might not want to collect on a morning when you're in a rush. In the event that you cannot collect enough saliva or are having trouble, you can chew sugarless gum or try pressing your tongue against the back of your teeth or yawning. If you just cannot get enough saliva, you can cap it and collect more the next morning. Saliva is actually very stable for up to thirty days. If you collect over the weekend, it is perfectly fine to mail it on Monday.

Some women will need more extensive testing of saliva for severe cases of adrenal imbalances. There is more information about adrenal problems in Chapter 5.

Tips for Obtaining Accurate Test Results

Before you take the test, you should find out when you should take the last dose of any hormones you're already taking. For example, if you take your BHRT twice daily, your doctor may have you take your nightly dose ten to twelve hours prior to your saliva collection. Some doctors have a patient take her last dose of hormones twenty-four hours before her saliva test. I prefer that women use their hormones as usual the day before they test, including the nightly dose.

If you are taking BHRT, you can contaminate your test if you're using hormone creams or gels, so make sure you haven't used them on your face or neck for at least one week prior to test day. (That doesn't mean you can't use them at all. Just apply these doses elsewhere, according to instructions.) If you do use creams the night before on other application sites, make absolutely sure you wash your hands thoroughly afterward.

Also, be careful of face creams containing herbal or anti-aging ingredients that might interfere with the saliva test. Though they do not affect your hormone levels, certain ingredients can interact with the extraction of hormones from the saliva. If there's any question in your mind about any product you're using on your face or neck, don't use the product for five days beforehand. You can also ask the saliva-testing lab about any product; just be sure to have the ingredient list handy when you call. Be aware that anything you touch, such as a hand towel, might still have hormone cream on it from the night before. Also make sure you change your pillowcase the night before the test day.

Certain supplements can affect the results of your saliva test. For example, herbal hormone balancing supplements such as phytoestrogens, a weight loss supplement called 7-Keto DHEA, adrenal supplements, and cortisol-reducing supplements such as phosphatidylserine, theanine, and Relora can alter results. Again, check with your physician or the saliva-testing lab if you are concerned.

Interpreting Results

The crucial point to remember is that you and your BHRT provider need to take into consideration your symptoms as well as your lab results when designing your treatment protocol. The numbers are very important, but because everyone is different, numbers can't possibly tell the whole story. What might be a perfect hormone level for someone else might not be perfect for you, which is why symptoms are such a crucial consideration. You can have symptoms of a deficiency or excess when your lab results are "normal." As with any other lab report, next to your hormone level you will find the expected "normal" ranges of the hormone based on age, menstrual status, and any hormones you are using. Even when your hormone levels fall within the normal range, if they are at the high or low end of the normal range, you may still need hormone therapy or dosing adjustments to resolve symptoms. If hormone levels look good but you have symptoms of an excess or deficiency, there must be something else going on; you may need further testing such as a thyroid panel, a fasting insulin test, in-depth adrenal testing, or neurotransmitter testing. Another thing you have to remember in interpreting hormone test results is that you can't consider only absolute numbers of each hormone individually. You also have to look at the ratio of each hormone level to the others, not only in the case of estrogens and progesterone, but also where adrenal hormones and thyroid hormones are concerned.

STEP 4: CORRECT IMBALANCES WITH BIOIDENTICAL HORMONES

Addressing Hormonal Deficiencies

Dosing Forms

Bioidentical hormones come in a variety of forms. In addition to the familiar pills and capsules, there are transdermal (which means through the skin) forms such as creams, gels, and patches. There are also sublingual (under the tongue) lozenges, troches that are placed in the cheek, sublingual drops, and even intravaginal suppositories for treating vaginal dryness and atrophy. Compounding pharmacies put bioidentical hormones in handy pumps or easy-to-measure syringes (no needles) for precise measurement. Hormones even come in pellets that can be implanted under the skin. The problem with pellets is that since they last about three months, you can't adjust the dose once they're implanted. I've seen a lot of women with hormone sensitivities, so it is very important to be able to change doses quickly. The pellets release a high level of hormone initially and then gradually decline somewhere between two to three months. Pellets are convenient but often expensive to have implanted. They are not my preference at all, however many physicians and patients do like them.

As I mentioned earlier, don't assume that any hormone product sold at a traditional pharmacy is synthetic or animal-derived. Some of these bioidentical hormones, such as estradiol patches and gels and progesterone capsules in a peanut-oil base, are available by prescription from traditional pharmacies in set dosages just as traditional HRT hormones are. The chart in Chapter 2 lists common hormone products and indicates which are bioidentical and which are not.

Many bioidentical hormones are prepared at compounding pharmacies. These pharmacies create formulations of hormones and other medicines customized for each patient according to doctors' specifications, permitting the doctor to adjust the dose to fit each patient's needs exactly. On the other hand, some bioidentical hormones are available without a prescription, including progesterone cream and DHEA. Estradiol, biest (a combination of estradiol and estriol), and testosterone all require a prescription.

Unfortunately, some opponents to BHRT want you to think that compounded hormones are not safe or that compounded hormones may not be reliable. Compounding pharmacies are regulated by each state's pharmacy board and by the Pharmaceutical Compounding Accreditation Board. The hormones they use are regulated by the U.S. Pharmacopoeia and the Code of Federal Regulations, which requires purity testing. The prescriptions filled at compounding pharmacies are not FDA regulated or FDA approved but do contain hormones that are FDA approved.

The obvious benefit is that your doctor can prescribe bioidentical hormones in individualized dosages and combinations with delivery systems that are not commercially available. Compounded prescriptions can also specify the creation of hypoallergenic creams and gels without the use of excipients and chemical preservatives.

Dosing Form Pros and Cons

Understandably, many women prefer the convenience of oral forms of BHRT, but there are important disadvantages to swallowing hormones. As you know, glands in your body secrete hormones directly into your blood stream. Hormones were never intended to go through your digestive tract before reaching their target tissues. When you swallow hormones, they must be digested and metabolized in your liver before they can enter your blood stream. This process is called first-pass metabolism, during which 90% of the hormones are converted to metabolites (by-products), leaving only 10% of the hormones in their original and proper forms. It's not ideal because these metabolites have different effects from those of the original hormones. For example, oral progesterone can be converted to metabolites that often cause very significant drowsiness, depression, and bloating in some women. And, of course, in order for you to get an effective dose, the BHRT practitioner has to prescribe as much as ten times the dose you actually need. For example, you have to take 100-200 mg of oral progesterone to get the same effects you would get from 20 mg of transdermal progesterone cream. I will say that many BHRT experts do prescribe oral progesterone and many women really do enjoy the side effect of drowsiness when taken at night. It is just not my personal favorite choice.

The biggest problems occur with oral estrogen. When estrogen undergoes the first-pass metabolism mentioned above, it stimulates the liver to produce triglycerides and blood-clotting factors as well as binding proteins that can affect levels of other hormone levels including thyroid. The greatest cause for concern associated with oral estrogen is the increased risk of blood clots. On the other hand, a recent study indicates that women who use estrogen patches have no higher risk of blood clots than women who take no hormones, and the researchers believe it is because the transdermally administered hormones don't pass through the liver.

Another problem with oral estradiol is that it rapidly converts to the estrogen called estrone. If the body doesn't process this form of estrogen correctly, it can increase the risk of breast cancer. Yet another issue is the fact that the binding proteins mentioned above can bind with other hormones, especially thyroid hormones; as we've learned, this binding can lead to a functional hormone deficiency, even when your body makes adequate amounts. That's the last thing you want when you're trying to get all your hormones balanced.

Comparison of Transdermal Estrogen and Oral Estrogen

Transdermal Estrogen	*Oral Estrogen*
• Lowers triglycerides • Lowers LDL (the bad cholesterol) • Decreases tendency toward clotting • Is less likely than oral estrogen to raise blood pressure • Has minimal impact on C-Reactive Proteins (inflammatory markers associated with cardiovascular disease) • Is twenty to fifty times more efficiently absorbed • More effective in managing weight and insulin resistance	• May increase triglycerides • Oral estradiol converts rapidly to estrone, which may be converted by the body into by-products that increase risk of breast cancer • Increases risk of blood clots • Increases Interleukin 6 (associated with numerous health problems) • Increases C-Reactive Proteins (inflammatory markers associated with cardiovascular disease) • Increases Sex Hormone Binding Globulin, Cortisol Binding Globulin, and Thyroid Binding Globulin, which makes these hormones less available

You have probably gathered that my personal choice in dosing forms is transdermal. Hormones applied transdermally are efficiently absorbed, and this absorption has been well demonstrated in research. I dislike sublingual (under the tongue) dosing because it is not possible to accurately monitor hormone levels with saliva testing, which is crucial to hormone balance. On a side note here, there are some labs and practitioners recommending women not use progesterone in the form of cream due to negative side effects. I must dispute this recommendation. Maybe these practitioners have noticed problems in patients taking excessive levels of progesterone cream such as 100 to 200 mg. (Most women feel great on 10-40 mg and have normal lab values.) I have heard one conference speaker state that transdermal progesterone causes elevated cortisol. Research has proved that progesterone cream lowers night time cortisol levels. In reviewing thousands and thousands of saliva tests over the past ten years, I have never seen the use of physiological dosing of progesterone cream, such as 20 - 30 mg, raise cortisol levels.

You also need to know that if you use transdermal hormones, blood testing will *not* measure the increase. Hormones are fat soluble and are carried by the red blood cells in the plasma - these are the free hormones that are bioavailable to the target receptor. Blood tests only measure hormones in the serum (the watery component of the blood after the cells have been discarded). You cannot accurately check to see whether your doses are correct using blood testing while on transdermal hormones.

Using Estrogen

If your saliva test shows that your estradiol level is low, you may need estrogen supplementation. Even if your test shows your estradiol at a low-normal level or less than optimal, you may feel better on estrogen. Of course, your BHRT specialist may try other approaches first. If you do need estrogen, there are some things you should know.

First of all, women normally produce at least three different kinds of estrogen: estrone (E1), estradiol (E2), and estriol (E3). (For a review on the three types of estrogen and the role estrogens play in the body, go back to Chapter 3.) They're all important for optimal health, but none should be used inappropriately. E1 and E2 are aggressive estrogens in that they have a proliferatory effect on hormone-sensitive tissues, such as those in the uterus and breasts. By proliferatory, I mean that they induce cells to multiply and divide. E3 is not believed to have this effect. In a process called differentiation, progesterone brings this multiplying of cells to a halt, allowing the cells to die normally. If proliferation goes unchecked, the cells can begin to proliferate wildly enough to become cancerous. Cancer is pretty much a matter of wild, uncontrolled, abnormal cell growth. Now you can see why it's so important that you have enough progesterone to balance your estrogen. I must point out here that there are numerous risk factors that increase breast cancer risk. Some BHRT treatment regimens call for estradiol as the only estrogen, but other practitioners may include estriol and estrone. A combination of estriol and estradiol is called bi-estrogen, or bi-est for short. Not surprisingly, a combination of all three estrogens is called tri-estrogen or tri-est. Tri-est was used in the early days of BHRT, but since your body converts estradiol to estrone, Tri-est is no longer preferred. The added estrone in Tri-est can be converted into metabolites (by-products) that can become carcinogenic. Using Tri-est is "old school" at this point. Estriol is sometimes used by itself, especially in women deemed to be at high risk for breast cancer or who have a history of breast cancer.

Estrogen Cream or Gel

Estrogen cream may be dosed once or twice daily. It may be estradiol only or biest, which contains estriol too. Doses are 0.1 mg and up. Dosages of estrogen cream and gel vary greatly according to the prescriber; I believe in conservative dosing because most women respond well to lower doses, and repeat saliva testing shows them to have achieved normal hormone levels. A typical dose would be 0.1 - 0.5 mg of biest once or twice daily. Estrogen cream is usually sold in a syringe or other dispensing device to make it easy to measure the correct dose. Compounding pharmacies can also combine several hormones in appropriate doses into a single cream, such as estrogen, progesterone, and testosterone. You can apply it to inner arms, inner thighs, neck, and abdomen, rotating application sites to prevent saturation of tissues. Never put estrogen on the breast tissue.

More About:

Applying Estrogen Cream: Choose a time of day that works best for you. Morning doses are preferred by some women. Apply after a bath or shower (after towel drying) rather than just before bathing. Evening doses can be applied when you're preparing for bed. Since hormone creams don't require refrigeration, you can keep them in the bathroom.

Dispense the amount the prescription label directs into your hand and rub the cream into the application site. Normally these sites include the inner forearms (from wrist to elbow), inner thighs, abdomen, and the back of the knees. Continue rubbing for a few moments to ensure penetration. Rotate the sites to avoid saturating the tissue in one area. Continual use in any single area may eventually saturate the hormone receptors there, reducing overall absorption. Keep in mind that any topically applied substance can remain on the skin for up to eight hours and be transferred to others by physical contact, so select application sites that will be covered by clothing. Also be sure to wash your hands before touching anyone or anything else. Please be sure you read this carefully: never apply estrogen to your breasts!

Creams prepared by compounding pharmacies will be dispensed in some sort of container that will make measuring easy. Often it will be a syringe with a cap (no needles) that displays units of measure so that all you have to do is push the plunger to the line indicating the prescribed amount. It is very simple and the compounding pharmacist should include instructions and/or be available to you by phone should you have questions.

Patches

If you receive estradiol-only (as opposed to Biest) supplementation, your BHRT practitioner may prescribe an estradiol patch to be changed once or twice weekly. For patches, I recommend the semi-weekly patch over the weekly patch because many women find that the once-weekly patch wears off too soon. Personally, I think the patch is very effective because it releases the estrogen evenly. Fluctuations in estrogen can cause hot flashes, and research is suggesting that these fluctuations are one cause of migraines. This even release is very effective and helpful in alleviating both of these symptoms. Just apply the patch to the buttock or to the abdomen, just above the pubic hair. The patches I prefer come in tiny sizes 1/2 inch wide. Others can be as large as Band-aids.

Estradiol patches are available from traditional pharmacies. Patch doses range from .014 mg (not very commonly used), to .025 mg, .0375 mg, .05 mg, .075 mg, and .1 mg of estradiol. I would say it is always best to start low if you have never used estrogen before. Most of the patients I have seen do well on the lower doses, and their saliva tests verify it. Other women require the highest level. For women already on high doses of HRT who are trying to switch to BHRT, it may be best to start at a mid-range dose.

There are two drawbacks to using the estradiol patches. Some women are sensitive to the adhesive. Bear in mind that each brand uses different adhesives, so the fact that you have a problem with one does not mean that you will have the issue with another. The other draw back is that the additional benefits of estriol are not included as with Bi-est.

More About:

Applying Estradiol Patches: Apply the patch to the buttock or lower abdomen, just above the pubic hair. Obviously, change the weekly patch once a week and the semi-weekly patch twice a week, preferably every 3 days for steady release. Make sure you remove the old patch before applying a new one. And remember, remember, remember never to use estradiol, estrone, or estriol without progesterone. Always use enough progesterone to balance estrogen to prevent estrogen dominance.

Intra-vaginal Estrogen

Estradiol, Biest, or Estriol creams can be used intra-vaginally for vaginal dryness that does not resolve with the normalizing of hormone levels. There are numerous estradiol receptors in the vaginal tissue, and often that tissue needs to be saturated directly with estrogen. Many women respond beautifully to Vagifem™, a bioidentical prescription estradiol tablet. It is used daily for ten days and twice weekly afterward. Women usually prefer this tablet to messy creams. Besides, some of the prescription estradiol creams have a mineral oil or petroleum base, which you may not want in such sensitive tissue. Be advised some creams prescribed for vaginal dryness or atrophy are conjugated equine estrogen (a non-bioidentical estrogen derived from pregnant mares' urine). Compounded creams would not have the mineral oil and would be a better option if you prefer a cream. Your compounding pharmacist can even put estrogen vaginal cream into a non-messy capsule. Actually, the same cream that your BHRT physician prescribes that you normally use on your arms or legs can be used intra-vaginally. You can do this by placing the designated dose on your finger tip and inserting it.

Oral Estrogen

Even though oral estrogen is not recommended for previously stated reasons, common dosing of estradiol is 1 to 2 mg. Oral Biest can range from 0.625 to 2.5 mg.

Estriol Only

Transdermal dosing of estriol can range from 0.25 mg to 0.5 mg once daily or every other day. Since estriol tends to accumulate in the skin, avoid excessive dosing. It can be applied to inner arms, inner thighs, face and neck, or abdomen, rotating application sites. Estriol can also be used intra-vaginally. Signs that you might be taking too much estriol are breast tenderness, bloating, water retention, and headaches.

Face Creams

And here's some good news - both progesterone and estriol discourage collagen breakdown and reduce the number and depth of wrinkles when applied to the face and neck. Who wouldn't want that? I use a special, very low dose of estriol and progesterone face cream mixed with other wonderful skin nutrients. Just remember not to apply hormones to your face for seven days prior to your saliva test. Simply choose another application site during this time.

Phytoestrogens

If lab tests show that you have low-normal (but still within the normal range) estradiol, sometimes phytoestrogens can help, and many healthcare providers often recommend their use. If your estrogen receptors just need a little nudge, they may work for you, but if lab tests indicate that you have a true estradiol deficiency, you will probably need some bioidentical estrogen. If you choose to use phytoestrogens, please consider the cautions presented in Chapter Two.

A Better Non-Hormonal Plant Based Option

For women with low-normal estrogen and women not able to take bioidentical estrogen, a viable option is black cohosh. There are numerous studies documenting black cohosh's effects on menopausal symptoms. Even better is that thus far research conducted has not found black cohosh to cause thickening of the endometrial lining of the uterus. Apparently it does not stimulate estrogen receptors and is technically not a phytoestrogen because its action is different. It binds to serotonin receptors rather than estrogen receptors. Physicians now prescribe medications like Prozac, which prolongs the life of serotonin, for hot flashes because it seems to alleviate them. Perhaps it is by binding to the serotonin receptors that black cohosh helps some women with hot flashes. (One study even found that black cohosh worked better for hot flashes than Prozac.)

Other research indicates that black cohosh is safe to use in breast cancer patients and may even inhibit tumor growth. Black cohosh appears to be safe for long-term use.

What to Expect While Using Estrogen

Whatever type of bioidentical estrogen you use, especially if it is transdermal, you may start to see the effects in a few days, but it may take as long as two weeks. If major symptoms like severe hot flashes aren't resolved in a month, the dose may need to be increased. Let your BHRT provider know. Signs that you might be taking too much estrogen are breast tenderness, bloating, water retention, and headaches.

Using Progesterone

Progesterone Cream

The most common starting dose of transdermal progesterone cream is 10-20 mg once or twice daily, but I have found that some women require doses as high as 40 mg or more. The need for higher amounts should be determined by lab values as well as clinical efficacy. A few women, especially those with estrogen levels on the lower end of the normal range, find that the typical starting dose of 20 mg once or twice daily is too much. Again, that perfect balance with estrogen is what we're after.

If you are still having periods, progesterone cream is best used according to your menstrual cycle. To determine the menstrual cycle timing, always count the first day of blood flow as Day 1. There are several ways to use progesterone.

One way to use progesterone is to start on Day 12 to 14 and continue through Day 26 or 28, which pretty well coincides with the luteal phase (the second two weeks of the cycle). (Some experts say to stop on Day 26. However, some women find that doing so does not control PMS on Day 27 and 28. Others find that if they do not stop the progesterone on Day 26, their periods will be late.) This approach of using the progesterone during the second two weeks of the cycle is used most often in younger, pre-menopausal women and in women desiring to conceive. Some perimenopausal women respond better to therapy when starting the progesterone on Day 7 and continuing until Day 26 to 28. With these varying suggestions, you and your provider can determine what is best for you.

Women whose cycles are irregular, and who consequently don't know what day of their cycle it is, can just start any time and adjust it to their cycles once they do start a period. If you find that your period comes before Day 28, just stop the progesterone and count the first day of your period as Day 1, starting over again. You can then start taking progesterone again on Day 7. You start the progesterone cream on Day 7, even if you are still bleeding. Post-menopausal women no longer having periods can either follow a three-weeks-on/one-week-off schedule or just take progesterone every day. For any of these situations, you will need to follow the BHRT physician's recommendation.

One of the latest recommendations for postmenopausal women is to take a one- day-per week break from all hormones. For example, use hormones every day except for Sundays. Patients seem to like this schedule best.

Over-the-Counter Progesterone Cream

Since progesterone cream is available over the counter, there are many brands available, providing doses of 20-25 mg. (As I mentioned earlier, it is also available by prescription in any dosage from compounding pharmacists.) I often run across web sites that say OTC progesterone creams are ineffective or that the creams actually contain no progesterone. In general, these web sites are simply wrong. There are many reputable brands containing United States Pharmacopeia (USP) progesterone, which is definitely effective. If the label doesn't list USP progesterone, don't buy it. Wild yam isn't really progesterone. One factor that varies quite a bit from one progesterone cream to another is the consistency of the cream base. Some bases are very thick or waxy and don't seem to penetrate very well, while others are very pure and very easily absorbed.

Even though progesterone cream is available over the counter, don't succumb to the temptation to treat yourself without saliva testing and the help of a BHRT specialist. Without testing, you might treat your symptoms successfully with OTC supplements only to find out later that you had other hormone imbalances that cause long-term problems. I had a patient, a knowledgeable nurse, who had treated herself with progesterone cream for years because she knew very well progesterone's bone-building properties. Imagine her frustration when she was diagnosed with osteopenia (low bone density, less severe than osteoporosis) after working so hard to keep her bones healthy. It turned out that her testosterone was low. Since testosterone deficiency correlates with loss of bone mass, she almost certainly would have benefited from testosterone supplementation as well if she had only known from proper testing.

More About:

Applying Progesterone Cream: Morning doses are best applied after a bath or shower (after towel drying) rather than just before bathing. Evening doses can be applied when you're preparing for bed. Since hormone creams don't require refrigeration, you can keep them in the bathroom. Dispense the amount the prescription label directs into your hand. Rub the cream into the application site. Normally these sites include the inner forearms (from wrist to elbow), inner thighs, abdomen, and the backs of the knees. Continue rubbing for a few moments to ensure penetration. Rotate the sites to avoid saturating the tissue in one area. Continual use in any single area may eventually saturate the hormone receptors there, reducing overall absorption. Keep in mind that any topically applied substance can remain on the skin for up to eight hours and be transferred to others by physical contact, so select application sites that will be covered by clothing. Also be sure to wash your hands before touching anyone or anything else.

Creams prepared by compounding pharmacies will be dispensed into some type of device that will make measuring the dose easy. Often it will be a syringe with a cap (no needles) that has units of measure so that all you have to do is push the plunger to the line indicating the prescribed amount. It is very simple and the compounding pharmacist should include instructions and/or be available to you by phone should you have questions.

Over-the-counter creams may come in jars, pump bottles, or tubes, which can make measuring the prescribed amount a little tricky. I would suggest that you check with your physician because what the product label recommends is a general dosage, and it may not be the amount the physician intends for you to use.

One nice added benefit of using transdermal progesterone is that using your breasts as application sites can help relieve discomfort associated with fibrocystic breasts and dense breast tissue. Check with you BHRT physician first.

Oral Progesterone

Recall that bioidentical hormones taken orally are metabolized through the gastrointestinal tract, and 90% are converted into metabolites. In the case of oral progesterone, this effect can trigger bloating, depression, and drowsiness. This loss of the original hormones in the digestive tract requires that dosing be much higher than is necessary with transdermal hormones. For example, most oral progesterone doses range from 100 mg to 200 mg.

There is a brand of progesterone capsules, called Prometrium, that is made by a pharmaceutical company. Prometrium contains peanut oil, so women with peanut allergies beware. Compounding pharmacies can also make progesterone capsules. Oral progesterone only stays in the body for four to six hours, but it can be compounded in a manner that makes it sustained-released. Many

BHRT physicians like to prescribe oral progesterone and get very good results for their patients with anxiety or insomnia.

Signs of Too Much Progesterone

Though your body never overproduces progesterone, it is possible to take too much supplementary progesterone. Fortunately, any symptoms of excess progesterone disappear when the dose is reduced to its proper level, and we know of no long-term adverse effects of supplemental bioidentical progesterone. As with any hormone, either excess or deficiency of progesterone triggers symptoms, sometimes even the same symptoms. Signs that you are taking too much progesterone include bloating, drowsiness during the day, increased hot flashes and wakefulness at night. If you take way too much progesterone you could also put on a little weight or have increased appetite. As I said, progesterone in the right quantity actually alleviates these symptoms, but as is so often the case, balance is the key.

Progesterone in Specific Situations

Seek medical advice for all specific conditions.

PMS and Cramps

Progesterone used days 7-28 as discussed above, is great for PMS and cramps. A teenager may need progesterone only during the last week of her cycle, usually Days 21 to 28. It would be wise to seek medical advice.

Women often ask whether they can use progesterone cream to treat PMS, even though they're using oral birth control. Used properly, natural progesterone shouldn't alter the effectiveness of birth control pills; however, I'm not aware of any research studies on the subject. Many health care practitioners do use progesterone cream to ease PMS symptoms in women on the pill, but results may not be optimal. We don't know whether progesterone can reach progesterone receptors in your cells when the receptors are blocked by molecules of the synthetic progesterone in the pill. At any rate, when using birth control pills you should use progesterone cream only *after* Day 14 to 16 of your cycle, once the pill has already blocked ovulation.

Addressing neurotransmitter imbalances can also reduce painful periods. Women with painful cramping are often low in serotonin and have an imbalance in norepinephrine.

Fertility and Miscarriage

Since progesterone is necessary for conception, for fetal brain development, and to prevent miscarriage, it can be used when trying to conceive. In fact, a woman who is deficient in progesterone may have difficulty becoming pregnant. Many practitioners find that women having trouble conceiving often succeed after starting progesterone supplementation. Women using progesterone for this purpose should use it from Day 14 through Day 26 to 28. Gynecologists and Reproductive Endocrinologists often prescribe intra-vaginal suppositories of progesterone for miscarriage prevention in women with a history of miscarriage. These suppositories are bioidentical. If you have had a miscarriage and have conceived again, have a discussion with your doctor about the use of progesterone.

Breastfeeding/Postpartum Depression

You can use progesterone while you're breastfeeding, according to your health care professional's directions; it has been shown helpful for postpartum depression. Unlike estrogen and testosterone, it isn't gender-specific, so it won't adversely affect babies of either sex. Babies are surrounded by very high levels of progesterone in the womb. During her third trimester, a woman makes about 300 mg of progesterone per day, compared to 4-24 mg per day during the luteal phase of the menstrual cycle. This high level of exposure to babies should attest to the safety of progesterone. Having said this, you still would not want to put progesterone on your skin where the baby could touch it.

Thyroid Medication

Women taking thyroid medication should be aware that progesterone deficiency or more specifically, a low progesterone-to-estrogen ratio could inhibit optimal thyroid function in the cells. Since thyroid hormones play such an important role in energy, mood, weight control, and many, many other vital processes, you don't want anything to impair your thyroid function.

Progesterone facilitates thyroid utilization by helping thyroid hormones get out of the blood stream and into cells, where they deliver their "messages" or perform their proper functions for that cell. Many people with adequate thyroid hormone levels experience functional thyroid deficiency, meaning that their thyroid hormone function is compromised such that they experience symptoms of hypothyroidism, sometimes even while taking thyroid medication. These symptoms include low body temperature, cold hands and feet, depression, low libido, poor concentration, and inability to lose weight, among others. Often these symptoms resolve when hormone imbalances like progesterone deficiency or cortisol excess are corrected.

Occasionally, progesterone supplementation helps a woman so much that she can reduce her thyroid medication, under medical direction of course. It is possible, though rare, for progesterone supplementation to help the thyroid so much that symptoms of *hyper*thyroidism appear, including heart palpitations, jitteriness, or headaches. If you experience such symptoms, your doctor should re-check your thyroid hormones and adjust your thyroid medication if necessary or adjust progesterone dosing. If symptoms of hyperthyroidism become severe, stop taking progesterone immediately and consult your physician.

Low Estrogen Symptoms

One of progesterone's most important functions is increasing the sensitivity of estrogen receptors, which means that your body has to have adequate progesterone in order to use the estrogen your body produces. This phenomenon explains why you can often eliminate low-estrogen symptoms like hot flashes and insomnia by raising your progesterone to a normal level, particularly when you aren't actually estrogen-deficient, only at the low end of the normal range.

Taking Testosterone

If your lab tests indicate a testosterone deficiency, it is very important that you not take a high dose. Men maintain about 3-10 mg of testosterone in their blood, but menstruating women make about a tenth of that, about 0.3 mg. After reading thousands of saliva tests, I've found that most women test in the normal range by using 0.1 mg to 0.25 mg, with a few needing 0.5 mg once a day or even just three times a week. So please be very careful of high doses of testosterone. I've seen many women prescribed one to two milligrams of testosterone cream, and there is no need for this excessive dosing. It will not make us chase our husbands around the house for sex; in excess, it's more likely to make us hairy and irritable. Common starting doses of transdermal testosterone are 0.1-0.5 mg. Apply it once daily in the morning, or three times a week, to the wrist or inner thigh. Rotate application sites daily. Testosterone can be compounded in with your other hormones. You can apply it directly to the clitoris one hour before having sex, just for fun. Signs that you may be taking too much testosterone include acne, increased facial hair, and irritability.

Reducing Elevated Hormones

If your hormone test shows that you make excess estrogen or testosterone, there are things you can do to lower those levels. One way to reduce functional estrogen or testosterone is to increase the levels of Sex Hormone Binding Globulin, or SHBG for short. You probably remember from Chapter 3 that SHBG is a binding protein that binds to estrogen, testosterone, and its metabolite, dihydrotestosterone (DHT), so increasing SHBG can bind up and reduce the functional level of these hormones. You can raise SHBG levels by eating more fiber and vegetables, reducing your intake of fat, eating flaxseed and isoflavones, or taking these in the form of supplements. In fact, we require zinc to manufacture SHBG. Losing weight can help if you're overweight. It's also important to make sure that you have an optimal amount of the thyroid hormone T3. Conversely, weight gain, stress, synthetic progesterone, alcohol, excess insulin, and a high-fat/low-fiber diet tend to decrease levels of SHBG. As we said, SHBG reduces functional levels of both estrogen and testosterone. Now we'll look at ways to deal with excesses of each hormone individually.

Elevated Estrogen

There are several supplements that can lower your estrogen if it's too high. For example, a supplement called indole-3-carbinol (I3C), from a compound occurring naturally in cruciferous vegetables, such as broccoli, Brussels sprouts, and cauliflower, exerts anti-estrogenic effects, which undoubtedly contribute to its ability to help prevent estrogen-dependent cancers. It exhibits potent anti-tumor activity via its regulation of estrogen activity and metabolism, such as blocking cell-cycle progression, triggering apoptosis (which is the removal of cells with damaged DNA, in which cancerous changes could occur, to make room for new cells), and reducing tumor invasion and metastasis. A number of in vitro and in vivo studies have found that I3C prevents development of estrogen-enhanced cancers, including those of the breast, endometrium, and cervix. By the way, you cannot eat enough broccoli to accomplish this. You have to use supplements.

Vitamin B6 helps women with excess estrogen by helping push estradiol molecules off of estradiol receptors in a timely fashion. The supplement calcium D-glucarate may also be helpful in dealing with excess estrogen. And don't forget good old progesterone. Since it opposes estrogen, make sure you're taking enough progesterone to balance your estrogen. Remember, it's very important that your progesterone-to-estrogen ratio is right.

Elevated Testosterone

If your saliva test shows that your testosterone is elevated and you are not taking testosterone, you need to bring it down. Since one of the most common causes of elevated testosterone and/or DHEA is insulin resistance, it is a good idea to check your fasting level of insulin if you test high for either one. Some doctors prefer to check Hemoglobin A1C in diabetic or pre-diabetic patients. Another preliminary way to determine whether you are insulin resistant is to divide your triglyceride level by your HDL.

TG to HDL Ratio:
> 4 Disease
> 3 Leads to Disease
< 1.5 - 2 Good
< 1.0 Ideal

For example: Triglycerides 120/HDL 45 = 2.66 which needs to be improved.

Fasting Insulin
> 15 Disease
> 13 Leads to Disease
< 10 Good
< 5 Ideal

If insulin turns out to be the culprit, you will need to work on this root problem. See Chapter 5 for information about insulin resistance and how to address it. A study published in *Fertility and Sterility* demonstrated that 1800 mg daily of an OTC supplement called N-Acetyl Cysteine, (N-A-C), lowered testosterone levels and reduced insulin resistance in Polycystic Ovarian Syndrome (PCOS) patients. Saliva test results in our practice have demonstrated its efficacy in testosterone reduction.

A prescription medication called spironolactone (Aldactone) can also reduce testosterone levels. Spironolactone appears to exert its therapeutic effects by interfering with ovarian testosterone secretion and peripheral testosterone activity. Spironolactone can be effective for the treatment of hirsutism (facial hair) in women with polycystic ovarian syndrome as well as idiopathic (cause unknown) hirsutism. Clinically, we do see that it certainly does bring the testosterone down. Talk to your BHRT provider about side effects related to Spironolactone that you should carefully consider. Dosing ranges are 25 mg to 100 mg once or twice daily. In almost every case, I would recommend a trial of the N-A-C and other insulin resistance supplements along with dietary changes first.

Switching from Oral Contraceptives (The Pill) to Bioidentical Hormones

Switching from the pill to BHRT shouldn't be difficult, but you will want guidance from your BHRT provider. Normally you just finish a pack of pills and start progesterone on Day 7 or Day 14 as suggested above. If you're using the pill to manage severe PMS, menstrual pain, or heavy bleeding, be sure to see the section on PMS and heavy bleeding in Chapter 6. You may want to use 200-400 international units of vitamin E with progesterone and other key supplements. Be aware that the heavy bleeding you experienced while taking the pill or before taking the pill is no indication of what you will experience when you stop taking it. After you go off the pill, it could be up to several months before your hormones get back to normal, so you may need to work very closely with your BHRT practitioner during the transition. Some women find that the small amount of synthetic estrogen they got from the pill really made them feel better. Therefore, once they're off the pill, they experience some low-estrogen symptoms. If that's you, hang in there. If you can get through one cycle without the pill by taking progesterone and some good nutritional supplements, you can have your saliva test and find out what your hormone levels are. Then you and your BHRT provider can develop a treatment protocol to address your low estrogen and any other problems you're having.

Maybe I should point out that bioidentical hormones are not effective birth control and are not prescribed as such. Take it from a mother of four.

Switching from HRT to BHRT

Switching from HRT to BHRT shouldn't be difficult either. Our patients do just fine on an estrogen, usually in patch form, with transdermal progesterone initially. Later the estrogen and progesterone could be compounded together. We often find that women who have been on HRT shouldn't start with the lowest dose of estradiol. Once you've been off the HRT and on the BHRT for four to six weeks, you can take a saliva test to see whether your estrogen and progesterone doses need changing. The same saliva test can evaluate your testosterone, DHEA, and cortisol as well.

Follow-up Care for Your Hormone Makeover

As we said before, after you start on BHRT you will need follow-up care. Many practitioners review the patient's progress in a follow-up visit approximately four to six weeks or no later than three months after they start BHRT. You will definitely need a repeat saliva test to determine whether your dosing is correct. Often, more testing is ordered, and therapy is adjusted. It may take a couple of adjustments to get your hormones balanced; it takes some patience, but you'll find it is well worth it. Paying careful attention to changes in your symptoms, taking good notes about them, and conveying that information to your BHRT practitioner can speed the process and improve the results. Once your hormones are balanced, you will need to be evaluated twice a year. You may find that your treatment protocol needs to be adjusted after periods of stress, significant weight gain or loss, or as endogenous hormone levels shift. Believe me, you'll be the first to know if something changes and you need to change your treatment plan.

The Next Component of Your Hormone Makeover

Now that we have you started on your hormone makeover, it's time to factor in and address the other critical elements of beautifully balanced hormones: your stress (adrenal) hormones, your thyroid function, and your insulin. We'll discuss all of it in the following chapter.

Chapter 5

RELATED HORMONES

STEP 5: MANAGE IMBALANCES OF RELATED HORMONES: ADRENALS, INSULIN AND THYROID

As if the effects of estrogen, progesterone, and testosterone weren't complicated enough, there are several other important hormones that interact with the reproductive hormones and each other in very complex and important ways. Specifically, you must have adequate and balanced levels of blood sugar, thyroid hormones, and adrenal hormones for optimal health. What makes diagnosing and treating hormone imbalance difficult is the enormous overlap of symptoms caused by shortages and imbalances of sex hormones, thyroid hormones, adrenal hormones, and the hormone insulin. But it's worth the effort to get it all sorted out because until you have optimal levels of all these substances, you can't feel your best or be in the best of health.

In the next three sections, we will cover the role of adrenal glands, insulin, and thyroid function one by one. In part one, we'll discuss the adrenal glands, the glands that respond to stress. We will list the symptoms of deficient and excess levels and explain how to address and correct these imbalances. Next we will focus on the hormone insulin in the same manner, followed by thyroid deficiency.

PART I
The Adrenals

These two small glands that sit on top of your kidneys are sometimes called the stress glands because they are responsible for producing hormonal changes that help us deal with emergencies and stressful events. But the adrenals actually play a bigger role in our physiology than just helping us handle stress.

The adrenal glands have two main parts: the adrenal cortex and the adrenal medulla. The adrenal cortex, the outer portion of the adrenal gland, secretes mineralocorticoids, glucocorticoids, and adrenal androgens. Androgens are considered masculinizing hormones. The hormones of the adrenal cortex are necessary to help us adapt to and handle stress. The adrenal medulla secretes epinephrine (adrenaline) and norepinephrine (noradrenaline). These hormones also mediate short term stress response. More detail about all of these momentarily.

If you feel well every day, your emotions are on an even keel, you have lots of energy, sleep great, wake up feeling refreshed, recover quickly from stress, and never have a problem with your weight, your adrenals are probably perfectly fine. If not, they may be somewhat overtaxed. We'll look first at the hormones secreted by the adrenal medulla, and then we'll look more closely at those secreted by the adrenal cortex because imbalances in these hormones are common and usually have powerful effects. Within each section, we'll discuss possible therapies for the imbalances, and then we'll discuss adrenal hormone testing.

Hormones Secreted by the Adrenal Medulla

The medulla, or inner part, of the adrenal gland produces the short acting hormones epinephrine (adrenaline) and norepinephrine (noradrenaline) to assist us in dealing with stressors of all sorts. We produce epinephrine in response to exercise, intense emotions like excitation, bursts of anger or embarrassment, or emergency situations. This rush of epinephrine allows us to handle the intense situation or emergency by increasing heart rate, dilating pupils, sending our blood supply toward muscles, brain, and heart. Any stored energy in the liver (called glycogen) is quickly converted to glucose. Some people also notice increased sweating or rapid breathing. Epinephrine and norepinephrine are familiar as the hormones that cause some of the physiological expressions of fear and anxiety in response to physical or mental stress or an emergency or scary event. These effects are short lived, meaning once we calm down excess levels clear from the body. Chronic excessively high levels of epinephrine and norepinephrine are associated with some anxiety disorders.

Hormones Secreted By the Adrenal Cortex

The adrenal cortex, the outer portion of the adrenal gland, uses cholesterol to synthesize all of the steroid hormones, including some of our progesterone, estrogens, androgens like DHEA and testosterone, mineralocorticoids, and glucocorticoids. These hormones influence chemicals in our blood, our bodies' metabolism, and certain body characteristics. We already know something about progesterone, estrogen, and androgens, but what in the world are mineralocorticoids and glucocorticoids? Mineralocorticoids are a class of hormones that help control blood pressure and balance the electrolytes like sodium and potassium in order to keep the blood slightly alkaline. Glucocorticoids, as cortisol or cortisone, promote normal metabolism such as protein catabolism (breakdown) and the release of fatty acids from adipose tissue (fat) to convert them to glucose. In more scientific terms, the primary role of cortisol is to promote gluconeogenesis, the vital process of converting fats and proteins to glucose. For the purpose of handling chronic stress, gluconeogenesis ensures that vital organs like the brain, heart, and muscles have energy. In urgent stress situations, cortisol assists epinephrine (adrenaline) in raising the heart rate and blood pressure. Glucocorticoids' role in stress response is to provide a sudden rush of glucose for alertness and to stimulate blood vessel constriction to increase blood pressure. They also serve as anti-inflammatory compounds.

Adrenal Androgens

Along with small amounts of progesterone, estrogens, and testosterone, the adrenal cortex also produces androstenedione and dehydroepiandrosterone (DHEA). Testosterone, DHEA, and androstenedione are all considered androgens. Let's take a closer look at DHEA since it's the most abundant steroid hormone in the human body.

DHEA

As you can see in the diagram below, DHEA is a precursor of (or contributes to the formation of) other hormones. About 40% of our estrogen and testosterone are made from the conversion of DHEA. Therefore, a deficiency in DHEA can trigger shortages of these hormones. DHEA levels decline with age anyway, dropping from its highest level in the second decade of life to about 50% of youthful levels by the time we reach the age of fifty. In our sixties, we typically produce only about 20% of what we did in our youth.

Hormone Cascade

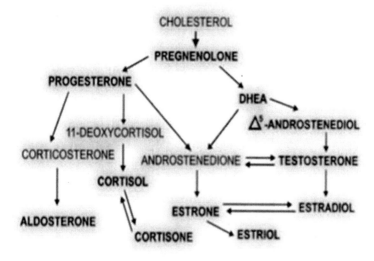

Aside from the age-related decline in DHEA that occurs normally, DHEA levels can drop to deficient levels in our younger years. So what causes a premature DHEA deficiency? In a word, stress. A hectic, stressful life with too many responsibilities takes a toll on hormones. Long-term, chronic stress can reduce the adrenals' production of DHEA, which I see very often in menopausal and perimenopausal women. It's extremely unfortunate since God intended the adrenals' contributory production of estrogens, progesterone, and testosterone to provide enough sex hormones to get us comfortably through menopause without experiencing extreme deficiencies in hormone levels. They're supposed to give us a soft landing, but since it's just not happening God's way, you may need DHEA supplementation.

The symptoms listed below have been correlated with or associated with lower levels of DHEA, though low DHEA may not necessarily be the cause of the condition/symptoms.

DHEA deficiency is associated with these problems:

- *Immune dysfunction*
- *Greater risk for certain cancers*
- *Heart disease in men*
- *Excess body fat*
- *Type 2 diabetic complications*
- *Chronic Inflammatory Disease*
- *Rheumatoid Arthritis*
- *Chronic back, neck, and shoulder pain*
- *Osteoporosis*
- *Neurodegenerative diseases*
- *Cognitive decline*
- *Depression*

Many symptoms of DHEA deficiency can also result from other problems, making diagnosis difficult. But here are common symptoms of DHEA deficiency:

- *Stressed feeling*
- *Intolerance of loud noises*
- *Moodiness*
- *Memory loss*
- *Constant fatigue*
- *Lack of stamina*
- *Poor abdominal muscle support*
- *Impaired immunity*
- *Dry eyes and skin*
- *Loss of pubic hair*
- *Low sex drive*

As with other hormones, DHEA has important roles in the body, including cardiovascular protection, protection of the brain, reduction of inflammation, promotion of immune function, and even with weight loss. Please see the list of DHEA actions.

Actions and Effects of DHEA

1. Protects the cardiovascular system by:
- *Strengthening the heart muscle*
- *Preventing blood clots*
- *Protecting against atherosclerosis*
- *Lowering cholesterol*
- *Reducing amount of atherosclerotic plaque (in animal studies)*

2. Protects the brain and central nervous system by:
- *Protecting against age-related deterioration of mental function*
- *Promoting brain function*
- *Protecting the brain from damage due to stroke*
- *Reducing risk of Alzheimer's*
- *Protecting brain from excess cortisol, which may prevent dementia*
- *Reducing inflammation*
- *Helping reduce lupus symptoms*

3. *Has antibacterial/antiviral properties/immune properties which improve immune function by:*
   - *Supporting immune system*
   - *Helping decrease allergic reactions*
   - *Possibly protecting against activation of HIV*
   - *Possibly fighting, in conjunction with melatonin, retroviral infection and anthrax toxin*
   - *Protecting against bacterial sepsis*
   - *Developing mature immune cells and enhancing antibody production*

4. *Additional properties of DHEA:*
   - *Decreases formation of fatty deposits*
   - *Increases bone growth*
   - *Promotes weight loss*
   - *Increases sense of well-being*
   - *Helps repair and maintain tissues*
   - *Diminishes allergic reactions*

Correcting DHEA Deficiency

Do not take DHEA supplements unless a saliva test indicates a deficiency or low-normal level. If you *know* you have a DHEA deficiency, please remember four extremely important things:

1) More is NOT better.
2) Most OTC DHEA oral supplements contain 25-50 mg per pill, which is a male dose. Rarely have I seen a woman who needed more than 10 mg. A woman should start with 5-10 mg if she takes it orally. If 25 mg does not bring up the DHEA level on your saliva test, you should consider using DHEA in cream form.
3) A transdermal dose of DHEA should be lower than an oral dose. A transdermal dose could be anywhere from .5 mg to 5 mg. Always start low and work up as necessary.

4) You need to monitor your DHEA level while taking DHEA supplements to make sure you don't overdo it.

Please be aware that, taken at night, DHEA might keep you awake.

Reducing Elevated DHEA

Excess DHEA is also frequently seen in women; it is generally triggered by insulin resistance, which will be discussed later in this chapter. However, stress can also stimulate excess DHEA production, as can polycystic ovarian syndrome (PCOS). Athletes tend to have higher levels of DHEA. Since it is an androgen, DHEA has some properties similar to those of testosterone, so symptoms of excess DHEA resemble those of excess testosterone: oily skin, acne, facial hair and irritability. If insulin resistance is the culprit in excess DHEA production, you need to improve insulin function. On the other hand, if your cortisol level is also elevated, reducing cortisol may reduce DHEA production to some degree. In any case, another way to bring down DHEA levels is to increase the levels of sex hormone binding globulin (SHBG), the protein coat we talked about earlier that can bind to DHEA. Increasing your fiber intake can increase SHBG levels, which, in turn, can lower DHEA. The use of the supplement NAC (N-Acetylcysteine) is also an effective approach.

Cortisol

Cortisol, an important hormone made in the adrenal cortex, is involved in proper glucose metabolism, regulation of blood pressure, insulin release for blood sugar level maintenance, immune function, and inflammatory response.

Although stress isn't the only reason why cortisol is secreted into the bloodstream, it has been termed "the stress hormone" because it's also secreted in higher levels during the body's "fight or flight" response to stress and is responsible for several stress-related changes in the body.

Functions of Cortisol

Cortisol plays a role in the metabolism of fats, proteins, and carbohydrates, so you wouldn't live long without it. And like other glucocorticoids, it helps direct your body's response to stress. Cortisol is, in fact, your body's main agent for dealing with stress.

In addition, when you're fasting, as when you sleep at night, cortisol prevents glucose from dropping too low. It stimulates the catabolism (breakdown) of proteins in your muscles and organs into their constituent amino acids so your body can quickly convert these amino acids to glucose, the brain's major fuel. This process is hard on your muscles and major body organs, but it keeps your vital central nervous system functioning at all costs.

Your cortisol level does not remain constant. Instead, cortisol production follows a diurnal (daily) rhythm. It should be at its lowest level between midnight and 2:00 a.m., when it slowly starts to rise to help us wake up and prepare for another stressful day. It normally drops rapidly between 8:00 and 11:00 a.m. and then continues to decline gradually throughout the rest of the day.

Cortisol helps regulate blood pressure and plays a part in other cardiovascular functions. It works in your immune system as well, mobilizing defenses against viral and bacterial infections. Cortisol is also, as mentioned earlier, an anti-inflammatory agent. We need adequate cortisol for normal functioning and for crisis response, but too much cortisol is, as I'm sure you've been hearing, very bad too. It's very important to get your cortisol level checked and deal with any imbalances as soon as you can. Just as with the other hormones, both excessive levels and deficiencies result in symptoms and health problems.

Chronic, Excessive Cortisol

Ok, I am sure you know by now that stress raises your cortisol level. This stress response is normal, enabling your body to operate optimally in an emergency. Short-term, small increases in cortisol for such emergencies provide quick bursts of energy for survival reasons, enhancing memory function, providing a temporary burst of increasing immunity, lowering sensitivity to pain, and helping maintain homeostasis in the body. Sounds great, doesn't it? However, problems arise when cortisol remains chronically elevated during prolonged periods of stress. Chronically elevated cortisol levels suppress the action of the immune system and predispose us to more frequent infections. We all realize that we are more prone to colds when we are under stress. Chronic elevation in cortisol, day after day after day, also breaks down muscle and bone, slows healing and normal cell replacement, and impairs digestion, metabolism, and mental function, among other things. Long-term elevation in cortisol is often called adrenal fatigue or hyperadrenalism. If the level is extremely high, it's diagnosed as Cushing's syndrome.

We think of stress as being caused by our life circumstances and events, and it often is, but physical stressors like illnesses, injuries, viruses, bacteria, and exposure to certain chemicals all stress our bodies too. Chronic pain and inflammation and even hormone imbalances can stress our bodies and push cortisol levels up. Athletes often have higher cortisol levels, as do women in the last trimester of pregnancy. Recent research has connected higher cortisol levels with estrogen deficiencies. And while levels of most other hormones decline with age, cortisol actually rises with age. Some researchers believe that many age-related diseases and problems result from a high cortisol-to-DHEA ratio. Some medications can increase cortisol as well. Unfortunately, eating high-glycemic foods like white flour and white sugar raises cortisol too. Worse, people with elevated cortisol tend to crave these very foods!

Symptoms or Conditions Related to Elevated Cortisol:

- *Insomnia/sleep disturbances*
- *Headaches*
- *"Tired but wired" feeling*
- *Stressed feeling*
- *Irritability*
- *Low libido*
- *Depression*
- *Food cravings*
- *Low serotonin (causes depression and carbohydrate cravings)*
- *Hormone resistance (meaning that the body is unable to properly use any or all of these hormones: thyroid, insulin, estrogen, testosterone, and progesterone, causing symptoms of deficiencies of these hormones)*
- *Thinning skin*
- *Loss of muscle mass*
- *Bone loss*
- *Heart palpitations*
- *Cardiovascular disease*
- *Breast cancer*

I've mentioned that stress really messes up hormone levels, mostly because cortisol (the stress hormone) interferes with the functioning of other hormones. Normal, short-term response to stress is good, and a normal cortisol level is essential, but long-term, high levels of cortisol cause a variety of serious problems. Excess cortisol depletes progesterone, causing symptoms of progesterone deficiency. High cortisol levels also block the function of thyroid hormones, causing symptoms of hypothyroidism. But we need optimal thyroid levels to clear cortisol from the body. On top of that, normal thyroid function is necessary to the *production* of progesterone in the first place, so high cortisol interferes with progesterone in two ways. More bad news!

High cortisol interferes with testosterone and insulin, possibly causing symptoms of testosterone deficiency and impairing blood sugar balance, leading to insulin resistance. Blood sugar imbalance, in turn, tends to cause weight gain, food cravings, and foggy thinking. Stress interferes with the release of neurotransmitters as well. In addition to enabling our brains to react to stimuli and make important mental connections, neurotransmitters have stimulatory and calming properties. Abnormal levels of neurotransmitters can, therefore, prevent clear thinking and normal reactions, as well as causing memory problems, depression, and irritability. Stress also depletes our bodies of the nutrients we need to keep our hormones in balance.

Symptoms and Effects of Excess Cortisol

The effects of chronically elevated cortisol are many, and none of them are good. Let's examine them more closely.

- **Tired but Wired Feeling:** This feeling is like you just drank several espressos, but you still feel tired.
- **Sleep Disturbances:** Since cortisol fosters alertness, elevated night-time cortisol disrupts sleep.
- **Low Libido:** Cortisol blocks testosterone from its receptors, which may explain the lower sex drive.
- **Food Cravings:** Cortisol triggers the release of fatty acids, glucose, and protein to provide energy during stress; cortisol remains elevated for a while after the stressful event ends in order to replenish fat stores by increasing your appetite. (Thanks!) So, chronically elevated cortisol encourages fat storage, in particular abdominal fat. High cortisol also stimulates something called neuropeptide Y, which turns on carbohydrate cravings and fat storage.
- **Abdominal Weight Gain or Obesity:** Since deep abdominal fat contains up to four times as many cortisol receptors as does superficial fat in other areas of the body, this type of tissue is more likely to respond to the cortisol it's exposed to. Unfortunately, it responds by storing more fat. What makes it

worse is that women with excess abdominal fat secrete more cortisol when stressed.

- **Blood Sugar Imbalances:** (such as hyperglycemia or insulin resistance). Cortisol blocks insulin from its receptors, causing the pancreas to produce even more insulin. Higher blood insulin levels lead to more fat storage as well as the normal issues associated with excess insulin.
- **Mood Changes:** One may feel irritable or stressed and elevated cortisol is even associated with depression.
- **Bone Loss:** Elevated cortisol inhibits the activity of osteoblasts, the bone-building cells. Cortisol is catabolic, which means it causes tissue to break down; therefore, elevated cortisol leads to bone loss. High cortisol also blocks calcium absorption in the gut and depletes magnesium, another mineral essential to bone health.
- **Increased Estrogen or Estrogen Dominance:** Cortisol stimulates aromatase activity. Aromatase is the enzyme that converts testosterone to estrogen. By the way, there is more aromatase in adipose (fat) tissue than other tissue.
- **Loss of Muscle Mass:** One loses muscle due to catabolism or excessive breakdown of muscle tissue.
- **Thinning Skin**: This problem is due to catabolism or excessive breakdown of skin.
- **Slow Wound Healing:** Cuts or scrapes take a long time to heal.
- **Impaired Immunity:** In particular, scientists have demonstrated that acute and chronic levels of stress and the resulting elevated cortisol are linked to upper respiratory infections, exacerbation of multiple sclerosis, and gastrointestinal disorders such as Irritable Bowel Syndrome.
- **Headaches:** Often tension related, these result from physical or emotional stress.
- **Heart palpitations:** These occur in response to anxiety.
- **Cancer**: Mounting evidence has linked stress, elevated cortisol, and cancer. A research paper published in *Psychoneuroendocrinology* in May 1996 reported that women with both early stage and metastatic breast cancer had significantly higher levels of cortisol compared with women without breast

cancer. Those with metastatic breast cancer had the highest levels. A more recent study in *Lancet Oncology* suggested that stress and depression result in immune system impairment and might promote the initiation and progression of some types of cancer.

- **Fluid Retention:** This annoyance is probably due to the stress effect on the mineralocorticoids, which are produced by the adrenals.
- **Low Serotonin Levels:** Low levels can trigger depression, carbohydrate cravings, and sleep disturbances.
- **Cardiovascular Disease:** Stress adversely affects multiple factors in heart diseases.
- **Hypertension:** In the *European Heart Journal,* a twenty-one year prospective study of 14,000 women and men indicated that chronic stress is an independent risk factor for cardiovascular disease, particularly fatal stroke.
- **Glycation:** Glycation is the binding of a protein molecule to a glucose molecule, forming damaged, non-functioning structures that accumulate in our collagen, corneas, brains, nervous systems, arteries, and vital organs as we age. Damage by glycation results in stiffening of collagen in skin and other tissues, leading to high blood pressure, wrinkles, and many other age-related symptoms. Arterial stiffening, cataracts, and neurological impairment are at least partially attributable to glycation. Chronic elevation of cortisol increases glycation.
- **Impaired Cognitive Performance:** Such impairment includes the atrophy of the hippocampus of the brain, affecting memory and recall. Excess cortisol inhibits short-term memory, so you forget things like where you put your keys. Evidence suggests that elevated cortisol may promote degeneration and death of neurons as well as decreased memory function in otherwise healthy elderly people. A study in *Neurology* found that people prone to experiencing high levels of stress had twice the risk of developing Alzheimer's disease compared to those who were not stress-prone. Other research has shown that people over the age of sixty-five who are physically fit are better able to

withstand stress and produce less cortisol than elderly people who are out of shape.

- **Reduced Human Growth Hormone:** Growth hormone levels affect muscle mass, lean body mass, the rate at which we age, etc.

- **Hormone Resistance:** Perhaps one of the most widespread negative effects of elevated cortisol is hormone resistance. High cortisol blocks other hormones from getting to their target cell receptors so that even when we have normal levels of estrogen, testosterone, insulin, and thyroid hormones, they may not be able to get where they are supposed to go. We may experience symptoms of deficiency while our blood or saliva tests show normal levels of these hormones. Elevated cortisol also depletes progesterone because progesterone opposes cortisol and is burned up in the process. Hormone resistance is a real problem when you're trying to get your hormones balanced. Since high cortisol can block your success, there is no way to completely resolve hormonal imbalance without addressing it.

- **Health Problems or Symptoms.** Elevated cortisol in the evening is associated with accelerated aging, higher breast cancer risk, sleep disturbances, and depression.

Cortisol's Interaction with Other Hormones

I am sure I don't have to remind anyone that stress, with its potential to elevate cortisol, interferes with hormone balance. We have touched on the affects of cortisol on the other hormones but here's a complete list of the interactions of cortisol with other hormones:

- **Progesterone.** Elevated cortisol competes with progesterone. It depletes progesterone levels, possibly leading to estrogen dominance. Estrogen dominance triggers symptoms of excess estrogen and overstimulates the endometrium, which is the lining of the uterus.

- **Testosterone.** Elevated cortisol blocks testosterone production and competes with testosterone at the DNA level, possibly leading to symptoms of low testosterone. However, since elevated cortisol tends to increase insulin resistance this can in turn lead to elevated androgens such as DHEA or testosterone in women.
- **Estrogen.** Elevated cortisol blocks estrogen in the brain, which can cause estrogen deficiency symptoms like hot flashes, even when estrogen levels are normal. Brand new research has found that estrogen-deficient women have higher levels of cortisol and thus more weight gain, especially in the abdomen. Recent research also suggests that estrogen supplementation can counteract the problem. To confirm the relationship between estrogen replacement and cortisol levels, researchers treated seven postmenopausal women not already undergoing HRT with a synthetic form of estrogen. After one month of therapy, these women, all of whom had previously had elevated cortisol levels, saw their cortisol levels decrease to levels close to those of premenopausal women.
- **Testosterone and Estrogen.** Elevated cortisol increases aromatase, the enzyme that converts testosterone to estradiol, sometimes causing elevations in estrogen.
- **DHEA.** Elevated cortisol can elevate DHEA. This is because DHEA responds in an attempt to lower the elevated cortisol. Early in the stress phase, the body produces excess DHEA in order to try to normalize the cortisol level. However, long term elevation of cortisol may lead to DHEA deficiency.
- **Insulin.** Elevated cortisol increases insulin resistance.
- **Thyroid.** Elevated cortisol causes resistance to thyroid hormones, especially the more active thyroid hormone, T3, thus causing symptoms of thyroid deficiency. It also reduces levels of the less active thyroid hormone, T4, which is supposed to be converted to T3. Excess cortisol can also cause T4 to convert to something called Reverse T3 instead of T3. Reverse T3 is nonfunctional, but when the pituitary gland measures T3 levels in our blood, it doesn't distinguish between regular T3 and Reverse T3, so it doesn't increase its output of Thyroid

Stimulating Hormone (TSH) to compensate. Therefore, lab results can look normal while we're experiencing a shortage of functional T3. Speaking of skewed lab results, high cortisol can block the pituitary's release of TSH so that test results fall in normal range.

Reducing Elevated Cortisol

There are a variety of ways to address elevated cortisol. Below are some of the supplements I have found clinically effective.

Phosphatidylserine

Phosphatidylserine, a phospholipid that forms an essential part of cell membranes, is a very well-researched supplement. Over more than ten years, studies have shown that it reduces elevated cortisol induced by physical or mental stress. In 2004, researchers concluded that phosphatidylserine mutes the impact of stress on the pituitary-adrenal system. Researchers have studied phosphatidylserine's protective effects on brain function and memory too. Naturally, it also helps these people sleep at night. On the other hand, it can also increase dopamine, a chemical that increases alertness, which in some people can interfere with sleep. Recommended amounts are 100 mg to 500 mg, one to three times daily.

Vitamin C

Vitamin C is the most important nutrient for adrenal metabolism and is essential to adrenal hormone production. The more cortisol your adrenals make, the more vitamin C you need. Vitamin C even works as an antioxidant within the adrenal cortex itself. And several studies show that vitamin C at various doses (500-1500 mg) reduces cortisol levels in people under various types of stress. Patients taking vitamin C also have lower blood pressure and report less subjective stress. Because vitamin C is water-soluble, it's rapidly excreted, so it's best to take it several times a day. For best results, take vitamin

C with bioflavonoids for better absorption. Buffered C is less likely to cause gastric disturbances.

Essential Fatty Acids (EFAs) Such As Fish Oil/Flax Seed Oil

Fish or flax oil helps stabilize insulin release, which is good in and of itself. This stabilization, in turn, reduces cortisol output. EFAs also decrease production of arachidonic acid (an unsaturated fatty acid found in most animal fats), which is good because excess arachidonic acids increase inflammatory responses, which tend to increase cortisol levels. EFAs from fish or flax seed oil suppress the production of inflammatory substances. Volunteers taking 7 grams of fish oil per day for three weeks released less cortisol in response to stress than they did before starting the fish oil regimen. Their heart rates and blood pressure did not increase as much, either. Seven grams may be a bit high for the average person. Common amounts range from 1500 to 4000 mg. Check with your physician if you are taking blood thinners since fish or flax oil can thin the blood.

Relora

Relora is a combination of magnolia bark and philodendron that a few small research studies indicate is useful in controlling cortisol. A large percentage of people in these studies found that Relora helped them relax without drowsiness, and in one study, 82% of people found it effective in controlling stress-induced symptoms like depression, anxiety, irritability, mood swings, concentration difficulties, and restlessness. 76% of those in a study of people who overeat in response to stress reported a decline in high fat/sugar/salt snacking. 74% of subjects in one study and 84% in another reported more restful sleep while taking Relora. No significant side effects were reported, but 24% of people in one study reported some initial drowsiness while 6% reported mild and transient stomach upset. In addition, two compounds found in magnolia bark have been identified as anxiolytic (anti-anxiety) agents. Unlike anxiolytics such as benzodiazepines, found in medications like Valium®, the magnolia bark compounds don't cause central nervous system depression, excessive muscle relaxation, amnesia, or physical dependence. Relora is often used at doses of 300-500 mg two to three times a day.

Theanine

Theanine is an amino acid found in green tea that is frequently used in stress management and adrenal support. Ironically, even though tea contains caffeine it can be calming, because theanine has an antagonistic effect on caffeine. It is best known for its ability to induce a state of relaxation. Theanine creates a sense of relaxation by stimulating alpha brain waves. The alpha brain waves promote a deep relaxed but alert state and improved mental clarity. Theanine improves memory and learning ability and can protect the brain from degenerative decline. Theanine is also involved in the formation of several neurotransmitters (brain chemicals) including gamma-aminobutyric acid (GABA) a very calming neurotransmitter that induces relaxation and a sense of well-being; dopamine, which promotes alertness and positive mood; and serotonin, which reduces anxiety and encourages normal sleep. It does not cause drowsiness.

Research on theanine has demonstrated many other interesting findings too. For example, it may be protective in regard to heart disease and cancer. Some animal studies indicate that theanine may lower high blood pressure. Other studies suggest that it prevents lipid peroxidation of LDL, the "bad" cholesterol. Lipid peroxidation is the process whereby free radicals "steal" electrons from the lipids in our cell membranes. This results in cell damage. By the way, this is why we need adequate intake of anti-oxidants such as vitamins C and E. Theanine has also been shown to protect against stroke and cerebral hemorrhage when used with green tea, and to protect the brain from damage during stroke-induced ischemia, a condition in which reduced blood flow results in the brain temporarily receiving too little oxygen. Theanine even appears to have anti-carcinogenic effects, making cancer-killing drugs more effective while reducing toxicity to normal cells.

The normal dose is 100-200 mg, taken two to three times daily as desired, with or without food, but if you're under intense stress, you can increase it somewhat. The Food and Drug Administration recommends limiting intake to 1,200 mg per day; however theanine has been shown to be safe and there have been no reports of negative reactions or drug interactions. It starts to work in half an hour or so and is effective for eight to ten hours.

DHEA

Supplemental DHEA can lower high cortisol, enhance the brain's resistance to stress-related changes, maintain cognitive abilities, and protect against age-related diseases. People with high cortisol who have a DHEA deficiency usually have no trouble taking DHEA. Please note that you should never ever take DHEA supplements unless you know your DHEA level is low or low-normal, as verified by saliva testing. Even then, you need to be very careful about dosage. Starting doses for women are 5 to 10 milligrams orally or 0.5 to 5 milligrams transdermally.

Ginkgo Biloba and Adaptogenic Herbs

Research has also demonstrated that Ginkgo biloba supplementation can reduce stress induced cortisol levels. Adaptogenic herbs such as ginseng, including Siberian ginseng, also more correctly known as Eleutherococcus senticosus, can help our bodies adapt to and handle stress. Several studies on another powerful herb called Rhodiola rosea have demonstrated effectiveness in combating both physically and psychologically stressful conditions.

Thyroid Hormone Medication

Normal thyroid levels help clear cortisol from your body. Obviously, you should take thyroid medication only if your blood test indicates a thyroid deficiency, and it is properly prescribed by your healthcare provider.

Hormone Balance

Proper levels of thyroid hormone, progesterone, estrogen, and DHEA play a role in cortisol balance.

Lifestyle Management

Exercise and other stress-reduction and relaxation measures help reduce excess cortisol. Simple carbohydrates increase cortisol levels; therefore, a low-glycemic diet helps keep cortisol down. However important a healthy lifestyle is, in my experience, you will also need certain supplements to successfully reduce your cortisol. For more about high-and low-glycemic foods, please see the section on insulin resistance to follow.

But what if your cortisol level is too low?

Adrenal Fatigue or Adrenal Exhaustion: Low Cortisol

Long-term effects of stress on adrenal hormone production can occur in stages. Often beginning with high cortisol coupled with high DHEA, it progresses to high cortisol with low DHEA, and winds up with low levels of both cortisol and DHEA.

The longer the chronic stressors persist, the worse the adrenal issues can become. In the early stages, cortisol levels can be too high, which can trigger a rise in DHEA, but your body can put out high levels of the stress hormones for only so long. So in the next phase of evolving adrenal fatigue, cortisol may rise and fall unevenly as the body struggles to balance itself and is challenged even further by caffeine, excess simple carbohydrates, and physical or emotional stressors. The adrenals can eventually become so overburdened and drained that they can no longer produce adequate amounts of DHEA. (Though DHEA typically declines with age, it should remain within normal limits for your age.) In more advanced stages, the adrenals are so exhausted from overwork that they no longer produce normal levels of cortisol either. This condition is sometimes called hypoadrenia or adrenal exhaustion. At its worst, when cortisol production is extremely low by medical standards, it is called Addison's disease.

Symptoms of Cortisol Deficiency:
- *Severe fatigue*
- *Allergies*
- *Stressed feelings*
- *Irritability*
- *Aches/pains such as muscle and joint pain*
- *Heart palpitations*
- *Sugar cravings*
- *Chemical sensitivities*
- *Low body temperature or any low-thyroid symptoms*
- *Hypoglycemic symptoms when missing a meal or eating sugar: irritability, shakiness, headache, and foggy thinking*

Managing Low Cortisol

I have to give credit to Dr. James Wilson for his work in establishing these protocols. I have met him and had the opportunity to speak at some of the same conferences. Clearly, he is the world's leading expert on adrenal function. If you have cortisol deficiency or cortisol levels that fluctuate abnormally during the day as demonstrated in a saliva test, his book, *Adrenal Fatigue; The Twenty-first Century Stress Syndrome*, is a must read.

Vitamin C

In the section on managing high cortisol, we talked about Vitamin C being the most important nutrient for adrenal metabolism; it is essential to production of all of the adrenal hormones. It is just as important to the health of adrenal glands *under*producing cortisol as those that are *over*producing cortisol because you have to have vitamin C to manufacture the adrenal hormones. Therapeutic levels of vitamin C are 1000 mg three times daily in combination with bioflavonoids.

Vitamin E

Because vitamin E is involved in at least six different enzymatic reactions in the adrenal cascade, high amounts of vitamin E are necessary for the adrenals to maintain high levels of steroid production, even under normal conditions. If your adrenal glands have been overtaxed for any length of time, you really need lots of vitamin E for recovery, and it must be a vitamin E high in beta-tocopherols. You will find this information on the product label. You may need as much as 800 mg a day for a minimum of three months to see an increase in your cortisol level.

Pantothenic Acid

Pantothenic acid, one of the B vitamins essential for the conversion of glucose into energy, is present in higher concentrations in the adrenal glands than anywhere else in the human body because production of adrenal hormones requires enormous amounts of energy. For adrenal rehabilitation you may need to take about 500 mg of pantothenic acid three times a day.

Magnesium

People with adrenal fatigue (and PMS) tend to be deficient in magnesium. This mineral is necessary for creating energy in every cell of our body. We also need it to produce the enzymes and energy required for normal adrenal hormone production. Magnesium is critical for the recovery process in people with deficient adrenal hormone production. Common recommendations are 400 mg to 800 mg of magnesium daily in divided doses. It may be best utilized when taken at night. Magnesium works best when taken along with other important adrenal nutrients especially vitamin C and pantothenic acid.

Siberian Ginseng

Siberian ginseng supports and rejuvenates adrenal function, increases resistance to stress, normalizes metabolism, regulates neurotransmitters, counteracts mental fatigue, raises and sustains energy levels, and increases physical stamina and endurance. It also fights depression, calms anxiety, improves sleep, diminishes lethargy, lessens irritability, and promotes a sense of well-being. Siberian ginseng also counters depletion of adrenal stress hormones, normalizes blood sugar, stimulates antibodies to bacteria and viruses, increases absorption of B vitamins, and helps the body retain vitamin C. No wonder Russian cosmonauts and Olympic athletes use this adaptogenic herb. Adaptogenic means that it helps the body handle or adapt to stressors.

Ashwagandha

Ashwagandha is also an adaptogenic herb that helps with inflammation and pain, protects the brain, and normalizes cortisol levels. It has been used to help boost thyroid hormone production too.

Adrenal Glandular Supplements

The action of adrenal glandular supplements is to support, fortify, and restore normal adrenal function. They are not replacement hormones but provide constituents for adrenal repair. As the cells of the adrenals recover, they can begin to produce normal levels of adrenal hormones once again. In my clinical experience, adrenal cortex supplements seem to be quite effective for strengthening the adrenal glands.

Licorice

Licorice root is another important herb for supporting adrenal function. It fortifies natural cortisone production, thereby slightly increasing circulating cortisol, and it prolongs the life of cortisol molecules. It can also ease the symptoms of hypoglycemia (low blood sugar) and raise blood pressure. Often people with exhausted adrenal glands have very low blood pressure, so licorice root really makes them feel better. Of course, if you have high blood pressure, you should not use it.

Natural Cortisol

Some people feel so bad and have such low cortisol levels that for a while they need to take very low doses of natural cortisol. A maximum total of 20 mg per day of hydrocortisone (another name for cortisol), marketed under the brand name Cortef taken in divided small doses can emulate the natural secretion of cortisol, giving the adrenal glands a rest so they can recover and start producing their own cortisol again. I have seen physicians prescribe dosing such as 1.25 to 5 mg, two to four times daily, typically with a higher dose in the morning and lower amounts later in the day.

Adrenal Hormone Testing

Be sure to request that your cortisol and DHEA be measured along with estrogen, progesterone, and testosterone when you take your saliva test. As with all hormone testing, remember to watch for low-normal and high-normal levels. You can test in the morning only, or for a more comprehensive test of adrenal function, you can test morning and evening. The best test is four times a day (called diurnal testing): first thing in the morning, at noon, around 4:00 p.m. and at night before bed. As we mentioned before, cortisol should be highest in the morning (but still within the normal range) and gradually decline as the day goes on, following what is called a diurnal (daily) rhythm. It begins to rise around 2:00 a.m. so that we will be awake and alert when it's time to get up. It should be at normal low levels by nightfall in order for us to sleep. High cortisol levels at night will certainly interfere with sleep. In women with severe fatigue and sleep disorders, the more comprehensive—even though more costly—testing is very important to diagnose problems that may not show up if the cortisol is only tested one time a day.

Concluding Thoughts on Adrenal Hormones

You can see that adrenal hormones are absolutely critical to our health and wellbeing. Chronically elevated, fluctuating, or low adrenal hormones precipitate symptoms. In addition, adrenal hormone imbalances can disturb the balance of the sex hormones, blood sugar, and thyroid hormones, causing symptoms in these categories. The point is that well-balanced adrenal hormones are essential to a truly complete and successful hormone makeover.

PART II
Insulin

Insulin, sometimes referred to as the sugar-processing hormone, is critical for glucose metabolism, storage, and maintenance. When we eat food, the digestive process converts carbohydrates into glucose, a simple sugar, which is absorbed into the blood stream. The pancreas releases insulin in response to rising blood glucose. Insulin then enters certain cells and triggers a set of events that causes the cells to absorb glucose from the blood. The hormone also helps other nutrients get inside the cells, including vitamins, minerals, amino acids, and fatty acids.

Our bodies' demands for fuel vary from moment to moment, but the brain needs our blood sugar level to remain stable. So getting the cells the energy they need without changing that level is a critical function—that's the role that insulin plays. Insulin signals the cells to absorb glucose from the bloodstream. The body monitors what we've digested, resulting blood sugar levels, and cell demands, and releases insulin in just the right amounts. That's why a healthy body is described as "insulin sensitive."

Insulin Imbalance

Carbohydrates are broken down into glucose, so when you eat too many of certain types of carbohydrates, like simple carbohydrates or high glycemic carbohydrates, the level of glucose in your blood increases dramatically, causing the pancreas to release a large amount of insulin to deal with it. This surge often lowers blood sugar too much, causing fatigue, irritability, depression, mood swings, memory problems, confusion, and low libido as cells are deprived of fuel. And because the body now needs more sugar to balance the excess insulin, it craves carbohydrates. When you then eat more carbohydrates, the pancreas puts out more insulin, causing the cycle to repeat itself. If left unmanaged, insulin imbalance can sabotage all efforts to balance your other hormones. And eventually this overproduction of insulin, along with other risk factors, can lead to insulin resistance, which means that cells become less sensitive to insulin. This insensitivity forces your body to produce yet more insulin to deal with glucose. Does this sound like a vicious cycle? Unfortunately, high insulin levels cause the body to store fat, which is why insulin is often called the fat storage hormone.

Insulin Resistance

Insulin resistance is the body cells' gradual loss of sensitivity to insulin. Every cell in your body has insulin receptor sites through which glucose enters the cells; if there is a surplus of glucose from excess carbohydrates not burned up by exercise, the cells become overloaded and won't accept more. The result is that the cells become resistant to insulin. As we've learned, our bodies respond by producing even more insulin, resulting in high levels of insulin, glucose, and other unabsorbed nutrients circulating in the bloodstream. Because many of its symptoms are similar to those of other conditions, insulin resistance can go unnoticed for up to forty years when serious complications begin to surface or the pancreas can no longer keep up with the demand for insulin. When the pancreas gives out, hyperglycemia (high blood sugar) occurs, and the diagnosis of diabetes often follows.

Some experts believe that 25% of Americans are insulin resistant, but how many more of us are in the early stages? Since insulin is a major hormone, it is critical in managing the minor hormones such as estrogen, testosterone, and progesterone. But the minor hormones affect insulin in turn. A decline or imbalance in the sex hormones in women can cause them to become increasingly intolerant of carbohydrates; therefore, the cells become less sensitive to insulin. Insulin resistance adversely affects fat metabolism because when cells won't absorb the excess glucose, the pancreas releases more insulin; now the liver has to convert the excess glucose into fat. These fat cells have a large number of glucose receptor sites, so these cells "want" sugar. When all those new fat cells don't get fed, women get tired or crave carbohydrates to feed them. It becomes a vicious cycle as women gain weight in a futile effort to feed more and more starving fat cells that never end up satisfied.

Symptoms of Insulin Resistance

Symptoms of insulin resistance may include fatigue (especially after meals), poor mental concentration, weight gain, abdominal (apple-shaped) obesity, edema, and an intense craving for sweets that may be very strong after a meal. Another important point to keep in mind is that excess insulin can drive up androgens, so if your androgens are elevated, you definitely need to check for and address insulin resistance.

Effects of Insulin Resistance

Weight Gain

It's unfortunate that so many people are unaware of the enormous contribution insulin resistance is making to the epidemic of obesity in this country. Most people suffering from insulin resistance are unaware since average blood testing may not show early stages.

Hormone Problems

Insulin resistance often leads to imbalances in adrenal, thyroid, and reproductive hormones. It is correlated with Polycystic Ovarian Syndrome (PCOS).

Cancer

Insulin resistance increases the risk of breast cancer, endometrial cancer, and other cancers as well.

Cardiovascular Problems

Research suggests that insulin resistance may be implicated in cardiovascular disease, leading to hardening of arteries, high blood pressure, high cholesterol, a bad ratio of good to bad cholesterol, and high triglycerides.

Aging

Apparently, insulin resistance accelerates aging in several ways. It increases the formation of free radicals, which damage cells of all types, and encourages the oxidation of fats. Since oxidation is the process whereby fats become rancid, obviously it's not a good thing. It is a partial explanation of the early aging of diabetics. It also reduces tissue elasticity, another unpleasant effect of aging. Insulin resistance has even been linked to Alzheimer's disease. What it all boils down to is that high levels of blood glucose and insulin are associated with accelerated aging and increased risk of premature death. On the other hand, normal blood glucose and insulin levels are associated with optimal health and longer life.

Diabetes and Other Metabolic Problems

Some are beginning to suspect that reactive hypoglycemia (low blood sugar), hyperglycemia (high blood sugar), and Type 2 Diabetes actually constitute a progression of insulin resistance. If true, Type 2 diabetes is really just insulin resistance at its worst. Some medical researchers are beginning to consider it simply early aging. Obviously, it's extremely important to maintain normal blood sugar levels to decrease the risk of developing diabetes as long as possible because many deleterious effects of high blood sugar accrue over time. In diabetics, tissues are injured when flooded by large amounts of glucose. Arteries, nerves, and the lens of the eye fall into this category, which is why uncontrolled diabetes can lead to blindness, neuropathy (nerve damage), circulatory problems, injury to arteries, renal disease, kidney failure, gangrene with consequent loss of limbs, and untimely death.

More About:

The Causes of Insulin Resistance
- *Genetic predisposition*
- *Diet (high-carbohydrate, high-glycemic, with excess simple carbohydrates)*
- *Obesity*
- *Sedentary lifestyle*
- *Smoking*
- *Stress*
- *Elevated cortisol*
- *Oral contraceptives*
- *Synthetic progesterone*
- *HRT*
- *Hypothyroidism*
- *Estrogen deficiency*
- *Elevated estrogen levels from overproduction or from excessive ERT*

Causes of Insulin Resistance

Research indicates that while some people are genetically pre-disposed, insulin resistance is largely a result of diet, lifestyle, stress, and imbalances in or deficiencies of other hormones. Remember back in the 1980s when we were told that the secret to weight loss was to cut way down on fats and proteins while eating lots of car-bohydrates? There were fat-free versions of everything. Didn't work out too well, did it? It turns out that a high-carbohydrate diet can encourage insulin resistance. In particular, simple carbohy-drates like sugar and starch—especially those high on the glycemic index, which cause glucose and insulin surges—foster it. Processed and refined foods, fats, and sodium can lead to insulin resistance. Overeating and obesity also contribute to insulin resistance. Certain mineral deficiencies have been implicated as well. You knew this was coming, but alcohol, tobacco, and lack of exercise increase your risk. Stress and the resulting elevated cortisol are risk factors and interestingly, either an excess of or deficiency in estrogen can lead to insulin resistance, including excess estrogen from ERT. Synthetic progesterone appears to be a problem as well, so oral contraceptives and HRT in general seem to encourage insulin resistance.

Since cortisol increases cells' resistance to insulin, the normal age-related increase in cortisol doesn't help. Cortisol also increases aromatase, an enzyme that converts testosterone to estrogen. The excess estrogen can cause estrogen dominance, which can, in turn, inhibit thyroid function. Hypothyroidism slows metabolism, and of course, slow metabolism encourages weight gain. Since being over-weight tends to increase insulin resistance, high cortisol encourages insulin resistance in two ways. Adequate thyroid levels are neces-sary to clear glucose from the body. Once again, we have another vicious cycle.

Testing for Insulin Imbalance

How can you tell whether you are insulin-resistant? Here are three red flags for starters: high blood pressure, high triglycerides, and high cholesterol. Even if you're young or slim, if any of these are elevated, it's time to test for insulin resistance. High blood pressure is particularly a red flag, and while blood pressure medication might control your blood pressure, it won't do anything for insulin resistance. Cholesterol problems may indicate insulin resistance, particularly if your triglycerides are high and your HDL is low. Here is an easy test you can do on your own to check this out. Divide your triglycerides by your HDL. For example if your triglyceride level is 140 and your HDL is 45, then $140 \div 45 = 3.1$. If your ratio of triglycerides to HDL is 2.0 or higher, you may be insulin-resistant. Ideal is 1 to 1.5. And more than nine out of ten women with acanthosis nigricans (dark, wart-like skin on the neck or armpits) are insulin-resistant. If you were ever diagnosed with gestational diabetes, have a family history of Type 2 Diabetes, or are very overweight, you should be tested. Also, women who tend to gain weight in the abdomen may have lower glucose tolerance and greater insulin resistance than those who tend to gain weight in the hips and thighs.

Here's a simple measurement you can make: without sucking in your stomach, measure around the narrowest part of your waist (approximately 2 inches above your belly button) and the widest place around your hips. If the ratio of your waist measurement to your hip measurement is greater than 0.8 (it's 1.0 for men), you're at risk for insulin resistance. But even if you're thin, don't assume you can't be insulin-resistant.

Everyone should be tested for insulin resistance periodically, but if you have any of the symptoms listed above, you should be tested sooner rather than later. The most helpful blood test is for fasting insulin level. The range is 1 to 27. According to Barry Sears, M.D., in *The Omega Rx Zone*, anything over 15 indicates insulin resistance, and 13 or higher indicates that insulin resistance is developing. He says a fasting insulin of 10 is good, and 5 is ideal. However, other experts think that fasting insulin over 8 indicates a problem. The optimal level of fasting insulin is *less* than 5. Another common test used by many physicians to assess for pre-diabetes is a blood test called hemoglobin A1c (HbA1c), which shows the average amount of sugar in your blood over the previous two or three months.

Addressing Insulin Resistance

Obviously, it's very important to lower your insulin levels. Doing so can promote fat loss, increase energy, enhance mental clarity, slow aging, lower blood pressure, improve cholesterol, and promote general good health.

Diet

Improving your diet is an obvious first step in reversing insulin resistance. Reducing calories and relying more heavily on foods low on the glycemic index (GI) will help a lot. The GI is a food-rating system based on the effect each food has on blood sugar. Foods that cause a rapid rise in blood sugar, and thus an excessive release of insulin, register high on the glycemic index. Low-glycemic foods, on the other hand, promote a slower, sustained release of glucose and insulin. Choosing foods with a low GI rating more often than those with a high GI may help you to:

- *Control your blood glucose level*
- *Control your cholesterol levels*
- *Control your appetite*
- *Lower your risk of heart disease*
- *Lower your risk of type 2 diabetes*

Non-starchy vegetables generally have low glycemic index levels. Proteins and good fats are also good choices for blood sugar and insulin control because they contain no carbohydrates; therefore, they register zero on the glycemic index. For more information, you can visit these sites:

Glycemic Research Institute at www.glycemic.com
www.mendosa.com/gilists.htm
www.southbeach-diet-plan.com/glycemicfoodchart.htm

Increasing your fiber intake will also help. See "Fiber" in the dietary supplements section below for more information. It's also important to include essential fatty acids (EFAs) in your diet to combat insulin resistance. You get them from avocados, eggs, flax seed, and cold-water fish like salmon. See the section "Essential Fatty Acids" for more information. Regular exercise also increases insulin sensitivity and promotes glucose uptake in the skeletal muscles. Besides changing your diet and getting more exercise, you may need to take some dietary supplements.

Dietary Supplements to Improve Insulin Sensitivity

Chromium

Chromium is a trace mineral that has remarkably positive effects on insulin and blood sugar, modulating blood glucose levels and reducing insulin resistance by as much as 40% while improving metabolism of proteins, lipids, and carbohydrates. It is the unique component of the blood-sugar-regulating molecule called Glucose Tolerance Factor (GTF). GTF works closely with insulin to facilitate the uptake of glucose into the cells, actually making insulin more effective. Research studies show that when plasma chromium levels are low, insulin resistance increases, and low chromium levels are directly related to high blood sugar, high insulin, and cardiovascular disease.

Chromium is excellent for people with hypoglycemia symptoms, including shakiness, irritability, mental fogginess, or headache after missing a meal or eating a high-sugar meal. It also helps Type 2 Diabetics lower their blood glucose levels. Though several types of chromium supplements are available, the most convincing research studied chromium picolinate and chromium polynicotinate. Take 400-1000 micrograms (mcg) per day in divided doses for best results.

A lot of research has been conducted on chromium to date. It has been shown to help lower cholesterol, increase longevity, and lower hemoglobin A1C levels. Many of these studies have been done on diabetics. One very impressive study done on a large group of people found that 1000 mcg of chromium improved hemoglobin A1C after four months and also lowered the fasting glucose levels.

Vanadium

Vanadium is another trace mineral that is very effective in the treatment of insulin resistance because it mimics insulin. According to research conducted at the University of British Columbia in Vancouver, sufficient doses of the vanadyl sulfate form of the mineral completely eliminated diabetes in laboratory animals. Human studies show similar therapeutic benefits in the treatment of diabetes. In order to derive the therapeutic benefits, many experts recommend 50 to 150 micrograms (mcg) per day used under a physician's care.

Cinnamon

When tested against forty-nine other medicinal plants, cinnamon appears to be one of the most powerful nutrients for improving glucose utilization. A study at a United States Department of Agriculture (USDA) research center found that chemical complexes in cinnamon play a role in preventing and alleviating insulin resistance and diabetes. A dose of 1, 3, or 6 grams of cinnamon per day reduced serum glucose, triglycerides, LDL cholesterol, and total cholesterol in people with type 2 diabetes, and scientists at Iowa State University found that some constituents of cinnamon activate the cell membrane's insulin receptors, increasing glucose uptake and therefore lowering blood glucose levels by 18-29% with doses of 1 gram and even more with doses of 6 grams.

Goat's Rue

An insulin-controlling agent used in medieval Europe to treat diabetes, *Galega officinalis* is rich in guanidine, a hypoglycemic substance (blood sugar lowering) that increases insulin sensitivity and lowers blood sugar and insulin. It has been shown to improve insulin sensitivity in both normal and diabetic people. In laboratory rats it produces a long-lasting reduction in blood sugar.

Alpha Lipoic Acid

Not only does alpha lipoic acid lower blood glucose, but it may also help stave off diabetes by decreasing the formation of the adipose tissue (fat) that increases the risk of diabetes. In animals, alpha lipoic acid has been shown to lower triglycerides, support the health of the pancreas, and cause weight loss. Possessing strong antioxidant properties, alpha lipoic acid also may protect against the adverse consequences of diabetes. It has even been used in Germany for well over two decades to treat diabetic neuropathy. R-lipoic acid is the more bioactive form. Dosing ranges of R-lipoic acid are from 50 to 150 mg per day.

Carnitine

Carnitine optimizes metabolism of fats and carbohydrates and promotes the sensitivity of cells to insulin. It encourages the storage of glucose and the lowering of blood sugar. A great deal of research indicates that carnitine is helpful in treating diabetes. For instance, it has been shown to lower hemoglobin A1C levels. Type 2 diabetics are often carnitine-deficient. Some consider acetyl-carnitine the best form to use. Average doses range from 500-1000 mg daily.

Coenzyme Q10 (CoQ10)

CoQ10 has been shown to help regulate blood sugar, lower blood pressure, quench free radicals, improve blood flow, lower triglycerides, and raise HDL levels, all of which would be important in preventing and managing the complications of diabetes. Animal studies have also shown that CoQ10 levels are depleted by diabetes.

Fiber

Along with its many other benefits, dietary fiber lowers and stabilizes blood sugar. One study found that diabetics who consumed 25 grams of insoluble fiber and 25 grams of soluble fiber dropped their blood sugar by 10%. Add fiber to your diet slowly to minimize digestive distress and disruptive effects on any diabetic medications you're taking. If you're diabetic, your medication may need to be reduced as your glucose levels drop, so consult your doctor before increasing your fiber intake or any blood sugar supplements for that matter.

Coffee Berry

Both of the two main nutrients in coffee berry, chlorogenic acid and caffeic acid, decrease and regulate the levels of glucose in the blood. Researchers have found that chlorogenic acid lowered blood sugar 15-20% and slowed the absorption of glucose in the intestines. This slowing of glucose absorption may reduce the body's insulin response, and lower insulin means less fat storage. Caffeic acid encourages cells to absorb sugar from the blood, which, of course, reduces the amount of sugar in circulation.

Essential Fatty Acids (EFAs)

EFAs help with some of the effects of insulin resistance and diabetes, reduce hypertension, and decrease triglycerides. Other benefits of EFAs include less weight gain, improved cognitive function, less inflammation, cholesterol reduction, and higher levels of HDL. EFAs are found in high doses in fish oil and flax seed oil supplements.

Magnesium

Magnesium may improve glucose levels. Diabetics are frequently magnesium-deficient.

The above constitutes only a brief list of the supplements that have been shown to improve blood sugar and reduce insulin resistance. Many, many other supplements and herbal formulas have positive effects on insulin resistance. Certainly one cannot take a long list of supplements for improved insulin utilization; therefore, supplement manufactures produce combination formulas of these and other effective nutrients that can do just the trick to help with blood sugar issues.

Medication

Physicians often put their patients with elevated glucose or elevated hemoglobin A1C levels on medication when necessary.

Metformin

Metformin is a medication from the class of drugs called biguanides. The exact mechanism by which biguanides work is not known, but the effects are well documented. Biguanides reduce insulin resistance in muscle cells and possibly other cells as well. They also reduce the release of glucose from the liver and stimulate the clearance of glucose. They also reduce the absorption of glucose in the small intestine after a meal. Because biguanides do not stimulate insulin secretion, they do not cause hypoglycemia (low blood sugar). They may help with weight loss. This and other similar medications are generally well tolerated, but some patients do not do well on them.

In summary, blood sugar balance is a key piece of a hormone makeover. Sex hormone imbalance can increase insulin resistance, and insulin resistance can create hormone imbalance. Insufficient thyroid hormone production can precipitate insulin resistance. Increased cortisol from chronic stress triggers insulin resistance. Once again, all three of these groups of hormones (sex hormones, stress hormones, and thyroid hormones) affect each other, demanding perfect balance.

Part III
The Thyroid Gland

Function of the Thyroid Gland

The thyroid gland, located in the front of the neck below the larynx (voice box), is vital to both men and women. Because the Greek root *hyper* means above and the Greek root *hypo* means under, hyperthyroidism is a condition in which the thyroid gland is overactive, and hypothyroidism is the condition in which the thyroid gland is less active than it should be. Women are much more likely than men to suffer thyroid problems, especially hypothyroidism, which often surfaces during perimenopause.

Levels of hormones secreted by the thyroid are controlled by the pituitary gland's thyroid-stimulating hormone (TSH), which, in turn, is controlled by the hypothalamus. The thyroid gland regulates the body's metabolism, thereby controlling the rate of function of every cell and gland in the body, including growth, repair, and metabolism. It also controls calcium balance throughout the body. The thyroid gland uses iodine to produce and secrete iodine-containing hormones called thyroxine (T4) and triiodothyronine (T3), along with the hormone calcitonin, which lowers the levels of calcium and phosphate in the blood, and promotes the formation of bone. The T4 and T3 hormones stimulate every tissue in the body to produce proteins and increase the amount of oxygen used by cells. Obviously, optimal function of the thyroid is vital to optimal health.

More About:

Thyroid Function:

There are several considerations in thyroid function. First of all, the thyroid must release normal amounts of thyroid hormones. Additionally, optimal amounts of thyroid hormones must be available to thyroid receptors and not bound by excessive amounts of Thyroid Binding Globulin. Further, proper conversion of T4 into T3 must occur. Then, the available T3 must be properly transported within the cells and the receptors must respond. Interferences in any of these steps can cause symptoms related to low thyroid function.

Thyroid Production- *requires nutrients such as tyrosine, zinc, copper, iodine and vitamins A, B2, B3, B6, C and E.*

Thyroid Binding- *excessive binding of available thyroid hormone can come from oral contraceptives, oral estrogens (synthetic or bioidentical) and estrogen dominance. This is because these substances increase Thyroid Binding Globulin which is a binding protein that makes less thyroid hormone available for use in the body. The nutrients vitamin A, D, Zinc and EPA/DHA help improve the ability of thyroid hormone receptors to bind to thyroid hormone.*

Thyroid Conversion- *or conversion of T4 to its active form, T3, requires the nutrients zinc, selenium, potassium, vitamins A, B2, E, tyrosine, iodine, growth hormone, testosterone, insulin, protein and melatonin.*

Thyroid Hormone Transport and Receptor Response- *thyroid hormones require a normal cortisol level, ferritin (iron stores) and vitamin D. Cortisol can be measured in saliva testing while ferritin and vitamin D levels are measured in blood. The vitamin D test to ask for is called 25- OH Vitamin D, and optimal levels of D are 60-80 ng/mL. Ferritin should be in the range of 90 – 110 ng/mL for optimal thyroid receptor function.*

A discussion of thyroid function is essential to the conversation about hormone balance for several reasons. First, in reviewing the symptoms of low thyroid function, you can easily see that many are also symptoms of sex hormone imbalance or adrenal imbalance. Therefore, it is important to evaluate the status of thyroid function if you have symptoms in this category too. Second, hypothyroidism and insulin resistance often occur in tandem, and their symptoms overlap as well. In fact, insulin resistance may even contribute to the development of hypothyroidism. Since thyroid hormones help clear glucose and insulin, reduced thyroid function can trigger insulin resistance. And insulin resistance is associated with poor nutrition, which also impairs thyroid function. It follows, then, that women with symptoms of hypothyroidism should also be evaluated for insulin resistance and vice versa. Third, the thyroid hormones influence and interact with the adrenal and sex hormones and neurotransmitters. Therefore, optimal thyroid function depends on the proper functioning of other body substances, including neurotransmitters, reproductive hormones, and adrenal hormones.

Let's look carefully at the effects of several hormones on the thyroid.

Effects of Other Hormones on Thyroid Function

Progesterone & Estrogen

Progesterone is necessary for thyroid hormone utilization because progesterone deficiency reduces the conversion of T4 to the more active T3. Therefore, a deficiency of progesterone can affect thyroid hormone function. Interestingly, T3 stimulates the production of something called Thyroid Inducing Factor (TIF), which stimulates production of progesterone by the ovaries at ovulation. As we see so often, a vicious cycle can form here.

A low ratio of progesterone to estrogen (estrogen dominance) also inhibits thyroid hormone function. In fact, because estrogen competes with T3 at the receptor sites, high levels of estrogen can trigger symptoms of thyroid deficiency. Additionally, oral estrogen increases the levels of Thyroid Binding Globulin which in turn binds up thyroid hormone and makes less thyroid hormone available to the body.

Cortisol

Excess cortisol interferes with thyroid function in several ways. It makes cells resistant to thyroid hormones and inhibits conversion of T4 to the more active T3. It can even cause the conversion of T4 into what is called "reverse T3." Reverse T3 competes with normal T3 but is non-functional. Most physicians do not check reverse T3 levels. What may be worse is that elevated cortisol reduces thyroid stimulating hormone (TSH) output from the pituitary gland. Elevated TSH levels mean your thyroid hormone production is low. So if high cortisol lowers your TSH blood test, then your tests can look normal while your thyroid function may be compromised. Frustrating and confusing, don't you think?

On the other hand, since a normal amount of cortisol is necessary for the thyroid to function efficiently, low cortisol levels can also cause functional thyroid deficiency. Functional thyroid hormone deficiency means that you have enough thyroid hormones, but they don't function properly at the cellular level. And since thyroid hormones help the body clear cortisol, people with low cortisol levels who begin taking thyroid medication may need to increase their cortisol levels to avoid the feelings of fatigue that often accompany cortisol deficiency.

So, you can see that there really are several key pieces to the puzzle in a hormone makeover, and optimal thyroid function is a major player. Since the most common thyroid hormone imbalance is hypothyroidism, we will examine it more closely.

Symptoms of Hypothyroidism

Symptoms of Hypothyroidism: Please note that each person may experience symptoms differently. Symptoms may include:

- *Weight gain*
- *Difficulty losing weight*
- *Exhaustion*
- *Lack of energy*
- *Excessive sleeping*
- *Sleep disturbances*
- *Low body temperature*
- *Intolerance of cold*
- *Cold hands and feet*
- *Decreased sweating*
- *Depression, mild to severe*
- *Memory loss*
- *Fuzzy thinking*
- *Difficulty following conversation or train of thought*
- *Slowness or slurring of speech*
- *Slowed reflexes*
- *Brittle nails or hair*
- *Anemia*
- *Hair loss*
- *Thinning or loss of sides of eyebrows*
- *Itchy scalp*
- *Dry skin*
- *Thinning skin*
- *Persistent cold sores, boils, or pimples*
- *Orange-colored soles and palms*
- *Joint and muscle pain*
- *Carpal tunnel syndrome*
- *Tingling sensation in wrists and hands that mimics carpal tunnel syndrome*
- *Low blood pressure*
- *Slow pulse*
- *Heart palpitations*
- *Blood clotting problems*
- *Bruising*
- *Elevated LDL (the "bad" cholesterol)*
- *Irregular periods*
- *PMS*

- *Diminished sex drive*
- *Infertility*
- *Miscarriage*
- *Breast milk formation*
- *Headaches*
- *Allergies (sudden appearance or worsening)*
- *Hoarseness*
- *Puffiness in face and extremities*
- *Constipation*
- *Calcium metabolism difficulties resulting in leg cramps or bone loss*
- *Insulin resistance*

Of course, you don't have to be overweight or manifest all of these symptoms to have less than optimal thyroid function. And you could have what is called subclinical or mild hypothyroidism and experience mild versions of these hypothyroid symptoms. You may even just feel fatigue or depression. So you should definitely be tested if you have any of these symptoms. Since the thyroid gland directly affects metabolism, many women with undiagnosed thyroid problems struggle needlessly with their weight. It's important to remember, though, that weight gain and difficulty losing often result from problems other than thyroid dysfunction, so weight gain by itself is not sufficient evidence of hypothyroidism. Other hormones, nutrition, and blood sugar balance are all important to weight loss and weight management. On the other hand, trying to lose weight without addressing thyroid deficiency could be futile. About 20% of menopausal women in the U.S. have been diagnosed with thyroid dysfunction, but sadly, recent studies suggest that millions more suffer from undiagnosed subclinical thyroid dysfunction. As we will see, this sad fact may be due in part to the interpretation of test results.

Thyroid Testing and the Interpretation of Results

There's a lot of controversy in the medical field regarding evaluation of thyroid tests and treatment of thyroid problems.

Most physicians will order a blood test called Thyroid Stimulating Hormone (TSH) to check your thyroid function. While many argue that only significant abnormalities should be treated, some experts believe that patients who test within the normal range but have many symptoms of low thyroid function need thyroid supplementation. Now, when I say "normal" I mean whatever the lab says is within the normal range. Obviously, interpretation of the lab results for thyroid function can mean the difference between getting therapy or not.

According to an article published in the August 3, 2002 issue of *The Lancet*, blood test reference ranges may not indicate the *optimal* level of thyroid hormone. When the pituitary gland detects that thyroid hormone levels are low, it releases TSH to signal the thyroid gland to produce more thyroid hormones. So, the lower your thyroid hormone production, the higher your TSH level will be. Therefore, TSH levels are one measure of thyroid gland function. According to some laboratories, a TSH level greater than 5.6 mU/L indicates hypothyroidism. However, a review of published findings regarding TSH levels indicates that TSH concentrations above 2.0 may indicate health problems related to inadequate thyroid hormone production and that people with TSH levels this high have a higher risk of developing hypothyroidism within twenty years. The authors of the above-mentioned study in *The Lancet* commented, "the emerging epidemiological data begin to suggest that TSH concentrations above 2.0 mU/L may be associated with adverse effects."

Another interesting study showed that thyroid hormone medication lowered cholesterol in patients with TSH levels of 2.0 to 4.0 but had no effect on cholesterol in patients with normal TSH levels between 0.2 and 1.9, suggesting that TSH values over 1.9 could indicate that thyroid hormone deficiency could be causing the excessive production of cholesterol. Even the American Academy of Clinical Endocrinologists recently suggested that physicians treat patients with TSH levels of 3.0 or higher, but it has not become a widely accepted practice, according to the web site www.aace.com.

Thyroid function test results should include your TSH number, and then usually just to the right on the lab report, you will find the reference range. Though the lab our office uses lists the normal reference range as 0.35 to 5.5, we follow an optimal range of .35 to 2.0 and consider treatment for women with TSH higher than 2.0. We normally see that women whose TSH levels are higher than 2.0 have hypothyroid symptoms and feel much better when treated. It's also important to know that HRT, oral contraceptives, or elevated cortisol can falsely lower your TSH.

What if you have lots of symptoms of hypothyroidism, but your TSH is less than 2.0? You still might have thyroid problems, which is why some experts believe in checking free T4 and free T3 levels along with TSH levels. The operative word here is "free," meaning bio-available. Remember in Chapter 3 where it was explained about bound versus free hormones? Those are the hormones that are bio-available, or useable, at the cellular level. Sometimes your TSH will be okay, around 1.8 for example, but levels of free T3 or free T4 may be a little low. According to one of our more progressive labs, normal levels of free T4 are 0.7-2.5, but the optimal range is 1.0 – 2.0. Normal levels of T3 are 2.5 to 6.5, with optimal levels 3.0 - 4.0. So, of course, when you have a thyroid test, you will want to ask that TSH, free T3, and free T4 be tested. You should also ask to have the TPO level checked. This measures thyroid antibodies which check thyroid auto-immune problems. Elevated TPO levels indicate that the thyroid is attacking itself, a condition that is called Hashimotos' Thyroiditis.

Optimal Thyroid Hormone Levels:

TSH: Optimal Range - .2 to 2.0, not as important as Free T4 and Free T3
Free T4: Optimal Range - 1.0 to 2.0 or middle to upper end of range
Free T3: Optimal Range - 3.0 to 4.0

As mentioned earlier, several factors can skew your thyroid test results. Elevated cortisol will decrease production of TSH, and your test level may look normal. So be sure to consider your cortisol level and possibly repeat your thyroid test once your cortisol is under control. Also as we said, oral contraceptives and HRT can falsely lower your TSH level and increase thyroid binding proteins. The result can be insufficient thyroid hormones in the tissues, while normal levels may circulate in the blood, giving normal levels on blood tests.

Even if all those numbers are in optimal ranges, you could still have what is called functional thyroid deficiency, meaning that the thyroid is producing normal amounts of hormones but those hormones are not functioning properly at the cellular level. This situation can occur because of imbalances in other hormones. High estrogen, low progesterone, or low androgens (DHEA or testosterone) can interfere with thyroid hormone function, as can either excess or deficient cortisol. In this case, correcting these hormone levels should restore normal thyroid hormone function. However, if blood tests indicate that you need thyroid supplementation, there are, again, differing opinions about treatment options.

Treatment of Low Thyroid

Often, healthcare providers prescribe the synthetic T4 hormone levothyroxine (Synthroid, Levoxyl, Unithroid) for hypothyroidism. But since T4 is one of two essential thyroid hormones, T4 alone does not always resolve the symptoms. The reason is that T4 is a long-acting thyroid hormone, but the liver must convert it to the short-acting, more active T3. Unfortunately, in many people the liver has trouble making the conversion of T4 into T3. Various factors can block this conversion, including poor liver function, lack of adequate minerals and other nutrients, high cortisol levels, and low progesterone-to-estrogen ratio. Therefore, many health care providers prescribe a combination of T4 and T3. A research study published in the May 2005 issue of the *Journal of Clinical Endocrinology and Metabolism* found that patients preferred thyroid treatment that included a combination of T4 and T3, rather than the usual levothyroxine (T4 only) treatment.

Other research trials have shown that treatment with a combination of T3 and T4 improved mood, energy, and cognitive function; such treatment also seemed to encourage weight loss. Medications that contain both T3 and T4 are Thyrolar, Armour Thyroid, Naturethroid, Westhroid, compounded dessicated thyroid and compounded sustained-release T4/T3 capsules. Many functional medicine physicians prefer desiccated thyroid therapy (Armour Thyroid, Naturethroid, Westhroid, compounded desiccated thyroid) since it also contains other active ingredients such as T1 and T2.

If you are taking a desiccated thyroid prescription be sure to take your blood test to check your levels four hours after your last dose.

Concluding Thoughts on Thyroid Issues

For the many women out there who have already researched low thyroid function and just "know" that you have thyroid problems in spite of "normal" test results, there is more to the story. Countless women do have untreated, subtle hypothyroidism and are struggling with the miseries of fatigue, weight gain, etc. Remember that there is more than one way to interpret the common thyroid tests; there are more sophisticated tests, and other hormone issues can create low thyroid symptoms by hindering the thyroid hormone function. My experience is that these hormone levels fluctuate, so it is worth repeating the tests if necessary. In addition, different doctors will have different interpretations, resulting in different approaches. It can be worthwhile to get a second opinion. Also, make sure that the adrenal hormones and sex hormones are balanced so that your hormone makeover will be complete.

Chapter 6

EXTRA HELP: RECOMMENDATIONS FOR GENERAL HEALTH AND SPECIFIC CONDITIONS

This section includes protocols I have found clinically helpful for specific symptoms. The suggestions are summaries and by no means exhaustive of all potentially effective therapies. And as I have suggested before, check with your own BHRT specialist or physician before commencing therapies.

In this book, I have already suggested the use of supplements. Their use is of vital importance to optimal health, of course, but in the matter of a hormone makeover, they are also required to balance hormones. Moreover, in regard to our overall health, the benefits of supplementation are well proven by research. At the very least, most people need to be taking a comprehensive multiple-vitamin and mineral formula and some form of essential fatty acids, such as fish or flax oil. Beyond the addition of supplements, we still have to eat right. An in-depth discussion on how to eat is beyond the scope of this book, and myriads of books on healthy diets are available. If you have not taken the time to read several, it will certainly be worth your time to do so. Please see my web site for some of my favorites. Nutritionists or Naturopaths can also help personalize a program for you if needed. Special tests called Functional Micronutrient Assay or NutriEval can detect cellular deficiencies of nutrients, anti-oxidants, and minerals.

I try to eat "real" foods that have been grown on the earth—not processed. I avoid hydrogenated foods, and I try not to eat foods with additives, preservatives, MSG, high fructose corn syrup, or that are high in sugar. I certainly avoid artificial sweeteners. Mounting evidence proves the importance of eating more fruits and vegetables. If you cannot do so, for whatever reason, you may want to consider fruit and vegetable supplementation. One of the most popular brands is Juice Plus+®. It is a whole food based product providing seventeen different fruits, vegetables, and grains. A large body of primary, peer-reviewed research has demonstrated improved immune function, improved circulation, reduced inflammation, and reduced oxidative stress in people taking this product. I have to rely on vegetable supplements because, in my busy life, I don't always get the recommended nine to thirteen fruits and veggies every day. I don't sell it, but I am sure you can easily find it on the internet. There are many other great greens, fruits, and vegetables supplements available too. There is no reason why we can't get enough with the resources we have access to today.

When it comes to buying supplements, you should be aware that all brands are not the same. Supplements come in four grades: veterinary grade, nutraceutical grade (found in many stores), medical grade (more pure, bio-available, in some better health food stores and direct marketing companies), and pharmaceutical grade—which have superior bio-availability and potency. Pharmaceutical grade supplement manufacturers follow the same strict production guidelines as pharmaceutical companies. The latter would be my preference for obvious reasons. Buying the cheapest versions of supplements may not result in optimal results. Beyond that, there is something else you should know; supplements that have not been thoroughly tested may even contain contaminants. One leading manufacturer recently had to recall its women's multiple vitamin after finding it contained high levels of lead. The bottom line is to buy the best quality supplements that you can afford from reputable sources.

Specific Conditions

STEP 6: ADDRESS SPECIFIC CONDITIONS SUCH AS PMS, BONE LOSS, AND BREAST CYSTS WITH INDICATED THERAPIES

For optimal results with your hormone makeover, you will most likely need to work on some specific symptoms or conditions. Here are some suggestions that I have found helpful to consider with your BHRT provider.

Hot Flashes/Night Sweats

Suggested Therapies:

50-75% of menopausal women complain of hot flashes and night sweats. They are really the same thing, but hot flashes are called night sweats if they happen when you're trying to sleep. The medical term for both is vasomotor symptoms. There are a variety of theories as to their exact cause, but here are some ways to get rid of them:

Estrogens: Estriol and estradiol both help relieve hot flashes, although estradiol more so. Sustained-released patches may work better than other dosing forms for some women, probably because it is fluctuations in hormone levels that seem to trigger vasomotor symptoms.

Progesterone: Progesterone is necessary to enable estrogen receptors to use estrogen. Therefore, if progesterone levels are low, you may not be able to use the estrogen your body is making. Thus, progesterone is all many women need to stop hot flashes and night sweats. For instance, in a research study, progesterone relieved hot flashes in 83% of post-menopausal women. However, if estradiol is very low, progesterone alone will not eliminate them. In fact, if estrogen is very low, adding progesterone can bring on or worsen symptoms of low estrogen, including vasomotor symptoms. This occurs due to progesterone's other role in balancing estrogen; it keeps estrogen from affecting the estrogen receptor as aggressively. So if you try progesterone cream and your hot flashes get worse, your estrogen levels may be very low. It does not mean you do not need progesterone; it just means that your estrogen level may be low.

Reduction of Cortisol: It's important to make sure that you don't have elevated cortisol. Many women find that they have hot flashes during stressful situations. Since cortisol causes hormone resistance, it can block estrogen in the brain, triggering hot flashes. Simple carbohydrates increase cortisol, which explains why some women get a hot flash when they eat sugar.

Fish Oil and Vitamin E: These two nutrients may help reduce the severity of hot flashes. A sudden drop in estrogen increases insulin production, and higher insulin levels increase production of two inflammatory substances: arachidonic acid and prostaglandin E2. There is some evidence that arachidonic acid and excess prostaglandin E2 trigger hot flashes. Therefore, fish oil or vitamin E may reduce hot flashes by helping counter these inflammatory chemicals in the body.

Phytoestrogens or Herbal Therapies: Phytoestrogens such as red clover, ground flaxseed, soy isoflavones, or the herb black cohosh can reduce the severity of vasomotor symptoms. They can be especially helpful for women whose estrogen levels are not extremely low but just on the low end of the normal range.

Watch Out for Foods That Trigger Hot Flashes: Of course, depending on the individual, there are various foods that can cause such a reaction. However, there are certain foods which are more prone to cause hot flashes, such as spicy foods, dairy products, very hot drinks or foods that are very hot in temperature, and acidic foods—especially acidic fruits, caffeine, sugary foods, and wine.

PMS

Suggested Therapies:

Progesterone: Progesterone is essential to reduce numerous PMS symptoms because PMS usually results from estrogen dominance. The importance of progesterone in managing PMS cannot be overstated and, as discussed in previous chapters, research supports the use of progesterone in the treatment of PMS.

Calcium and Vitamin D: Calcium and vitamin D are vital to PMS prevention because ovarian hormones are very involved in the metabolism of calcium and vitamin D (as well as magnesium), according to a research study published in the April 2000 *Journal of the American College of Nutrition*. Estrogen regulates calcium metabolism and intestinal calcium absorption, triggering fluctuations across the menstrual cycle. Researchers reported that disturbances in calcium regulation underlie pathophysiological characteristics of PMS. Furthermore, the evidence to date suggests that women with premenstrual symptoms during the luteal phase (last two weeks of the menstrual cycle) have underlying calcium dysregulation as well as vitamin D deficiency. Researchers have found enough similarities between the symptoms of PMS and the symptoms of calcium deficiency to determine that PMS represents the clinical manifestation of a calcium deficiency.

It's hardly surprising, then, that many research studies have shown that calcium helps prevent PMS. One such study published in the August 1998 issue of *The American Journal of Obstetrics and Gynecology* found that within three menstrual cycles, calcium supplementation effected an overall 48% reduction in total PMS symptom scores. The researchers compared the benefits of calcium to taking Prozac (an antidepressant) and Xanax (an anti-anxiety pill) for its effect on mood and depression and concluded that calcium was equally as effective for overall PMS relief and calming effect, at a lower cost and without the potential side effects. Other clinical trials in women with PMS have also found that calcium supplementation alleviates most mood symptoms.

A research study published in a 1994 issue of the journal *Headache* suggests that vitamin D and calcium therapy should be considered in the treatment of women who suffer with premenstrual migraines and PMS. The recommendation resulted from research showing that a combination of vitamin D and elemental calcium greatly reduced headache attacks as well as other premenstrual symptoms within two months of beginning therapy. Commonly used doses are 500-1000 mg daily of calcium. Be sure to ask your doctor to check your vitamin D level. You may need from 2000 to 10,000 units daily of supplemental vitamin D3 to get your vitamin D to an optimal level of 60 to 80+ ng/mL.

Magnesium: Magnesium is important for hormone production and metabolism and is essential for the proper use of calcium and vitamin D. Magnesium deficiencies have been noted in women with PMS, and it's even possible that chocolate cravings are related to low magnesium levels since chocolate (especially dark chocolate) is a natural source of magnesium. Estrogen enhances the body's utilization of magnesium. However, if estrogen levels are high or there is estrogen dominance and magnesium intake is less then optimal, estrogen-induced shifts of magnesium can lead to muscle spasms, migraines, and other PMS disorders. In one study serum levels of magnesium were inversely related to the serum level of estrogen.

A study published in the November 1998 *Journal of Women's Health* found that a daily dose of 200 mg of magnesium reduced premenstrual fluid retention within two menstrual cycles. In the second month, there was a reduction of symptoms of a form of PMS, called PMS Hyperhydration (PMS-H), associated with weight gain, swelling of extremities, breast tenderness, and abdominal bloating.

A study in the March 2000 journal of *Women's Health and Gender Based Medicine* reported that taking 50 mg daily of vitamin B6 in conjunction with 200 mg daily of magnesium for one menstrual cycle significantly reduced anxiety-related premenstrual symptoms like nervous tension, mood swings, irritability, and anxiety. Commonly used doses are 400-800 mg daily of magnesium in the form of chelate, glycinate, or citrate.

Zinc: Zinc deficiency was noted in PMS patients in a study conducted at the Department of Obstetrics and Gynecology, Baylor College of Medicine. Also, copper levels were found to be higher during the luteal phase in PMS patients compared with those of control subjects. The researchers concluded that zinc deficiency occurs in PMS patients during the luteal phase and that the elevated copper further reduces the availability of zinc in PMS patients. Too much copper can cause serious mood problems. As an added bonus, zinc also helps with premenstrual acne. Commonly used amounts range from 15 mg to 25 mg once or twice daily.

Vitamin B6: Since your liver needs vitamin B6 to break down and properly deactivate estrogen, vitamin B6 supplements can help lower excessively high estrogen levels. Deficiency of this vitamin may play a role in exacerbating imbalances in neurotransmitters and thus contribute to depression and mood swings. And since vitamin B6 helps in the metabolism of carbohydrates and proteins, adequate levels of vitamin B6 may reduce food cravings. Data also suggest that B6 may help women who suffer premenstrual dizziness, vomiting, impaired mental performance, and social withdrawal. In May 1999, researchers reviewing nine published research trials studying a total of 940 PMS patients concluded that up to 100 mg/day of vitamin B6 likely benefits women suffering PMS and premenstrual depression. All B vitamins work best when taken together in a vitamin B complex. Common doses are 25 mg to 50 mg twice daily.

Vitamin E: Vitamin E appears to reduce PMS as well. Suggested amounts are 200 IU to 400 IU once daily.

Note: A high quality women's multiple vitamin and mineral supplement may include therapeutic levels of all of these key PMS nutrients so that you don't have to buy numerous individual supplements.

Fatty Acids: Prostaglandins are hormone-like chemicals that control various bodily functions. There are pro-inflammatory prostaglandins and anti-inflammatory prostaglandins. According to research, women with PMS may have abnormal prostaglandin excretion (or imbalance) that may play a role in PMS. The anti-inflammatory prostaglandins promote smooth muscle contraction and blood vessel dilation, both of which are essential to the normal menstrual cycle. Supplementation with fatty acids can maximize the production of anti-inflammatory prostaglandins while suppressing pro-inflammatory prostaglandins. In two clinical studies, supplementation with omega-3 fatty acids reduced symptoms associated with PMS, including cramps.

Gamma-linoleic acid (GLA) is a long-chain polyunsaturated fatty acid found in evening primrose oil and borage seed oil. Like levels of omega-3 fatty acids, levels of GLA are abnormal among women with PMS. GLA can reduce some of the symptoms of PMS, even when other therapies fail. A large research study published in the *Journal of Reproductive Medicine* found GLA highly effective in treating premenstrual depression and irritability, breast pain and tenderness, and fluid retention. The study also suggested that women with PMS should consider taking other nutrients known to increase utilization of GLA. These nutrients include vitamin C, vitamin B6, magnesium, zinc, and niacin.

Dietary Improvement: Reducing carbohydrates, animal fat, sodium, dairy products, and caffeine can reduce PMS symptoms.

Chasteberry: Chasteberry has medicinally active components that induce the pituitary gland to produce Luteinizing hormone (LH). As we know, LH stimulates ovulation, triggering progesterone production during the luteal phase (Days 14-28) of the menstrual cycle. A 1998 research study found that chasteberry offered significant relief to women suffering from PMS, especially breast tenderness, cramping, and headaches. And in 2001, the *British Medical Journal* reported that more than half of the women taking chaste tree fruit extract (chasteberry) had a 50% or greater improvement in PMS symptoms (with the exception of bloating). The German government's Commission E, which evaluates herbal remedies prescribed in conventional medical practice in Germany, has approved chasteberry for menstrual irregularities, breast pain, and premenstrual complaints. CAUTION: WOMEN WHO ARE PREGNANT OR MIGHT BECOME PREGNANT SHOULD NOT USE CHASTEBERRY. Also, women taking hormone therapies of any kind, antidepressants, or dopamine-receptor agonists should consult a clinician before trying this herb.

Neurotransmitter Treatment: It is not uncommon for physicians to prescribe antidepressants called SSRIs to women with PMS. These medications inhibit the clearance of serotonin, thus making more of it available. Serotonin is an important neurotransmitter that is involved in the regulation of mood, especially depression. Some women do well on these medications but others often prefer a natural solution.

The supplement tryptophan is a precursor of serotonin that is sometimes used by physicians to treat depression by increasing the amount of serotonin naturally produced. The use of tryptophan has been shown to significantly reduce symptoms if administered during the luteal phase, which is the last two weeks of the cycle (day 14-28). Similarly, the supplement 5-hydroxytryptophan, or 5-HTP, may help relieve symptoms by increasing the production of serotonin. Although 5-Hydroxytryptophan has not been studied in PMS, it has been studied in the treatment of depression.

Neurotransmitter metabolite testing can serve as an invaluable tool for detecting such imbalances in PMS. If you have a neurotransmitter evaluation, you should take your test during the time of your worst pre-menstrual symptoms. For more information on neurotransmitter testing see www.mybrainchemistry.com or www.neurorelief.com.

By the way, it is important for women dealing with PMS not to ignore it. Yes, I know the symptoms may only last a few days each month but sadly they just come right back next month taking a toll on our relationships and life in general. Not only that, but the underlying hormonal imbalances can lead to other problems if left unattended. Moreover, one research study found that women with PMS are more likely to have menopausal symptoms.

Dysmenorrhea (Cramps)

Suggested Therapies:

Progesterone: Progesterone deficiency may be associated with higher levels of inflammatory prostaglandins; therefore, progesterone usually helps with menstrual cramps.

Vitamin E: Vitamin E has been shown in several studies to significantly reduce menstrual pain and blood loss. It works by inhibiting synthesis of the inflammatory prostaglandins that trigger the pain. Since women with dysmenorrhea have been shown to produce eight to fourteen times more of these inflammatory hormones, it makes sense that vitamin E helps them. Trials on vitamin E for cramps have used 200-500 IU. Some trials have used this supplement only for a few days before the onset of menstruation and for the first couple of days of bleeding with effective reduction in pain.

High-fiber/Low-fat Diet: Several studies have found that high-fiber/low-fat diets reduce menstrual pain.

Fish or Flax Oil: The omega-3 fatty acids in fish oil have anti-inflammatory effects. Omega-3 supplements have been shown to relieve dysmenorrhea, likely by affecting the metabolism of prostaglandins and other factors involved in pain and inflammation. It may require a dosage of 2000 IU daily.

Magnesium: Studies suggest that magnesium supplementation may be helpful for dysmenorrhea. A 6-month, double-blind, placebo-controlled study of 50 women with menstrual pain found that treatment with magnesium significantly improved symptoms.

Acupuncture: Acupuncture caused complete cessation of menstrual pain in 86% of the women in one study.

See the above section on PMS for additional information.

Menorrhagia (Heavy or Prolonged Bleeding)

Suggested Therapies:

Progesterone: Progesterone addresses estrogen dominance, which can cause heavy bleeding. Clinically, I have found progesterone very helpful in reducing heavy periods and menstrual blood clots.

Estrogen Metabolism Nutrients: The estrogen-metabolism nutrients such as I-3-C and B6 discussed in the section on breast cysts in this chapter may also reduce heavy periods.

Thyroid Hormones: Check thyroid hormone levels because an underlying thyroid deficiency can cause heavy periods.

Vitamin A: One research study found that women taking vitamin A experienced a 93% improvement in menorrhagia.

Vitamin E: A recent research study published in the *British Journal of OB/GYN* found that vitamin E, used a few days before a period, greatly reduced pain and flow.

Vitamin C + Bioflavonoids: Taking vitamin C with bioflavonoids has been shown to reduce flow and increase iron absorption.

Fish or Flax Oil: These may also reduce heavy bleeding.

Note: Make sure your doctor orders blood work to check to see if you are anemic if you are having very heavy periods. Low iron levels will certainly affect your energy levels.

Low Iron/Anemia

Suggested Therapies:

Heme Iron: Heme iron is a source of highly bio-available nutrients including iron, vitamin B12, and trace minerals. Heme iron is bound to hemoglobin and myoglobin and is the most efficiently absorbed form of iron. In fact, your body absorbs up to 35% of heme iron, compared to 3% of non-heme iron. Examples of non-heme iron supplements are ferrous sulfate and ferrous fumarate, which sometimes cause side effects such as gastrointestinal upset, constipation, nausea, flatulence, and diarrhea. Heme iron also contains other substances that promote healthy blood cells, including B12 and folic acid. Your local health food store should also have highly absorbable, non-constipating iron formulas. Vitamin C helps you absorb iron, so make sure you take good amounts.

Folic Acid and B12: In some cases, additional folic acid (800 mcg) and vitamin B12 sub-lingual lozenges (1000 mcg or more) may be necessary. Use methylcobalamin (a type of Vitamin B12).

Testosterone: Testosterone can markedly increase red blood count, so if you're testosterone deficient, this should be addressed.

A blood test, called an anemia panel by some labs, shows the factors associated with low hemoglobin levels, such as B12 or folate deficiency. Low iron is a separate problem from B12 or folate deficiency, but all can cause anemia. It is also important to test ferritin level because this is your iron stores. Hypothyroidism is another contributing factor in anemia.

Benign Breast Cysts, Fibrocystic Breast Disease (FBD)

Suggested Therapies:

Progesterone: As discussed in detail in chapter 3, researchers have demonstrated the effectiveness of progesterone cream in treating benign breast cysts. You need to ensure that your progesterone-to-estradiol ratio is correct; you should have one hundred to five hundred times as much progesterone as estradiol.

Thyroid Hormones: Evaluation and appropriate therapy can help address FBD. Researchers have linked breast abnormalities, including FBD, to hypothyroidism. It is postulated that treating thyroid problems will reduce the risk of FBD and ameliorate the symptoms. Hypothyroidism can cause overproduction of such hormones as LH, FSH, and prolactin. Almost half of the women in one small study reported total relief after daily treatment with 0.1 mg of the thyroid medication levothyroxine (Synthroid), and patients with elevated prolactin had normal levels after treatment with thyroid hormone. Other research has also found lower T4 levels in women with benign breast cysts.

Evening Primrose Oil: Several European studies have demonstrated the effectiveness of evening primrose oil in the treatment of breast pain and benign cysts; 13% of all British surgeons and 30% of British breast surgeons surveyed in 1990 recommended evening primrose oil.

Iodine Therapy: A review of three clinical studies showed that sodium iodide, protein-bound iodide, and molecular iodine affected clinical improvements in FBD of 70%, 40%, and 72%, respectively. See www.optimox.com

Fiber: Fibrocystic Breast Disease is apparently linked to constipation; women having fewer than three bowel movements a week have a four to five times greater risk of having FBD than women having a bowel movement each day. Of course, fiber helps.

Reduction of Methylxanthines: Caffeine, theophylline, and theobromine are methylxanthines found in tea, coffee, cocoa and soft drinks. They stimulate breast tissue to overproduce cellular products such as fibrous tissues and cyst fluid. Some studies show that avoiding methylxanthines can improve FBD symptoms by as much as 97%.

Improved Estrogen Metabolism: Optimal estrogen metabolism is important because estrogen stimulates the hormone-sensitive tissue of the breast and uterus. While a certain amount of stimulation is normal and necessary, overstimulation followed by a chain of events can cause cancer. So we want to make sure that estrogen does not stay too long on the receptor sites, is metabolized into forms of estrogen that are less stimulating to the breast tissue, and is properly cleared from the body. As I've said before, progesterone is essential to balance estrogens and to change estrogens into their less aggressive metabolites.

Besides progesterone, several nutrients assist in proper estrogen metabolism. Vitamin B6 pushes estrogen off of the receptor sites in a timely fashion. Fiber binds to estrogen metabolites and pulls them out of the intestine before they can be reabsorbed into the bloodstream, and probiotics increase elimination of inactivated estrogen metabolites via the large intestine. Indole-3-carbinol (I3C) occurs naturally in cruciferous vegetables such as broccoli and cauliflower and exhibits potent anti-tumor activity via its regulation of estrogen activity and metabolism. It also blocks cell cycle progression, triggering apoptosis (normal cell death), and the reduction of tumor invasion and metastasis. I3C exerts anti-estrogenic effects, which undoubtedly explains why it helps prevent estrogen-enhanced cancers. A number of studies have found that I3C prevents development of estrogen-enhanced cancers including those of the breast, endometrium, and cervix.

More About:

Research on I-3-C has shown it may:

- *Protect the genomic structure of DNA*
- *Convert dangerous estrogens (16-alpha-hydroxyestrone) that cause the development of abnormal cell colonies to safer forms of estrogen (2-hydroxyestrone) that prevent the development of abnormal cells*
- *Block estrogen receptor sites on the membranes of breast and other cells*
- *Restore p21 suppressor gene function*
- *Induce apoptosis (proper cell death) of cells*
- *Protect cells against the toxic effects of pesticides and other environmental pollutants, including dioxin*
- *Slow the propagation of abnormal breast and prostate cells*

Depression

Suggested Therapies:

Normalization of All Hormone Levels: Hormones have profound effects on mood. Depression is associated with both estrogen deficiency and estrogen excess. Deficiencies in thyroid hormones, especially T3, and androgens (DHEA and testosterone) often induce depression. Either cortisol deficiency or cortisol excess can also be the culprit in depression, as can progesterone deficiency. Remember that excess cortisol can block the actions of other hormones, resulting in functional deficiencies even when lab tests show normal levels of the other hormones.

B Vitamins: The B vitamins, especially vitamin B6, are essential for the production of neurotransmitters that affect mood.

5-Hydroxytryptophan (5-HTP): 5-HTP is converted to serotonin and raises levels of endorphins, which are "feel good" neurotransmitters. Some studies have found 5-HTP as effective as Prozac, Paxil, and Zoloft.

SAMe: SAMe is believed to address depression by increasing the synthesis of neurotransmitters dopamine, serotonin, and norepinephrine which are crucial to normal mood, behavior, and emotion.

Fish Oil: Fish oil increases serotonin and dopamine; dopamine encourages mental focus and emotional satisfaction.

Test Neurotransmitters: Consider testing neurotransmitters through a special urine test. See the web site of the lab that offers this test:
www.neurorelief.com
www.donnawhitehormonemakeover.com
www.mybrainchemistry.com.

Insomnia

Suggested Therapies:

Progesterone: Progesterone normalizes sleep patterns and is relaxing because of its effect on GABA, a neurotransmitter that has a very calming effect. Progesterone also lowers night-time cortisol levels and reduces night-time awakenings.

Estrogen: Estrogen reduces the time it takes to get to sleep and increases the amount of REM sleep we get.

Melatonin: Melatonin deficiency as we age is a very common cause of sleep problems.

Cortisol: Cortisol-reducing supplements are helpful if cortisol is elevated.

5-Hydroxytryptophan (5-HTP) or Tryptophan: 5-HTP reduces time required to fall asleep, decreases awakenings, improves REM sleep by 25%, and increases stages three and four of deep sleep.

Blood Sugar Stabilization: If you have a tendency to be slightly hypoglycemic, work on stabilizing your blood sugar. A drop in blood sugar triggers a release of adrenaline and cortisol, which stimulate the brain, triggering alertness. Eating a protein snack and/or taking chromium before going to bed will probably help.

There are many conditions that are related to or caused by hormone imbalances. The use of hormones and the correcting of hormone imbalances are absolutely vital, but bear in mind that other modalities are almost always necessary too. For example, you can take hormones and supplements but if you don't eat a good diet you may not have optimal results. If you eat right, take your BHRT and supplements but you do not take time to get adequate rest and sleep or even play, your hormone makeover will not be as good as it could be. There are women who will need to seek counseling or other medical therapies for their optimal health and wellness. There may be other important testing that you should do such as neurotransmitter testing, bone turn-over testing, or estrogen metabolism testing. The point is, there are many pieces to the puzzle. Don't over look a single important piece related to your health.

Chapter 7

BONE BUILDING

The bones are highly sensitive to hormonal changes. During puberty, when hormone levels surge, they stimulate bones to grow rapidly as teenagers grow into adults. Thus, it is not really surprising that in later years, as hormone levels decline, the bones become vulnerable once again.

Definition

Osteoporosis is the condition in which loss of bone mass and deterioration of bone structure lead to bone fragility, thus increasing the risk of fracture. More prevalent in women than in men, its incidence increases with age. At least ten million Americans have osteoporosis, and many more have a milder form of bone loss called osteopenia. The most common fracture sites associated with osteoporosis are the spine, hip, and forearm. Hip fractures cause approximately 50,000 deaths each year, and 50% of Caucasian-American women over seventy are expected to suffer a spinal compression.

General risk factors for osteoporosis:

- *Deficiencies of vitamin D, calcium, magnesium, or any other bone-building co-factors, usually resulting from poor diet*
- *Bulimia or anorexia*
- *Excessive protein consumption*

- *Heavy alcohol consumption*
- *Excessive caffeine consumption*
- *Smoking*
- *Lack of exercise*
- *Excessive exercise*
- *Extremely low (below 15%) percentage of body fat*
- *History of osteoporosis in mother*
- *Delayed puberty*
- *Long-term amenorrhea (lack of menstrual cycles)*
- *Hormone deficiencies*
- *Other endocrine disorders*
- *Postmenopausal status, whether occurring naturally or resulting from chemotherapy or removal of ovaries*
- *Advanced age*
- *Elevated blood acids*
- *Long-term use of corticosteroids or other medications*
- *Gastrointestinal disorders or use of antacids that interfere with mineral absorption*
- *Thyroid disorders*
- *Kidney disorders*
- *Bone cancers or other malignancies*

Testing for Bone Loss

Dual-energy x-ray absorptiometry (DEXA), the standard test for bone density, uses a small amount of radiation to measure bone density in the spine, hip, or wrist, the most common sites of osteoporotic fractures. A peripheral version of the DEXA, or single-energy x-ray absorptiometry, can be used to measure bone mineral density in the forearm, finger, and sometimes the heel. Urine tests can also measure the biochemical markers that indicate the amount of bone turnover. Though they do not measure actual bone mass and cannot directly indicate whether you have osteoporosis, your doctor may run these tests in between your yearly or biannual DEXA test since they are useful for evaluating the success of therapy. As always, be sure to get a copy of your lab results for your file.

The DEXA measures bone density based on average bone density of a large sample of healthy 20-29 year-olds. Normal bone density is defined by a T-score of between -1.0 and +1.0. The World Health Organization defines osteoporosis by a measurement of bone-mineral density that is 2.5 standard deviations below that of a healthy young person. T-scores between −1.0 and −2.5 indicate osteopenia, a lesser degree of bone mineral loss.

Understanding the Bone-building Process

The first step in learning how to manage, prevent, or reverse (yes, I did say reverse) bone loss is to understand the bone building process. In bones, as in all living tissue, cells die off and new cells are created in a process essential for bones to grow strong and remain healthy. Mass and density define bone health. Before your body can build new bone tissue, it must first remove the old bone cells in a process called resorption in order to initiate new, healthy bone formation. Bone loss occurs when resorption outpaces formation, also called mineralization or remodeling.

Bone Composition

Bones are composed primarily of the nutrients collagen, glycoproteins, and hydroxyapatite. Collagen, a fibrous protein, forms the largest component of the three. 35% of bone's mass is composed of a collagen matrix, or latticed protein, which gives bone its strength. Glycoproteins are carbohydrates and proteins that re-enforce collagen, and hydroxyapatite consists of calcium, phosphorous, and lesser amounts of several other minerals. Together, collagen, glycoproteins, and hydroxyapatite are the mortar that binds to the minerals in order to form bone in a process called mineralization.

Osteoclasts and Osteoblasts

The two major types of cells involved in this bone remodeling process, osteoclasts and osteoblasts, work together to perform the bone remodeling process. First, osteoclasts travel through bone tissue, removing old bone and leaving small, jagged spaces behind. This action spurs osteoblasts to deposit new bone in these spaces, so you can see that osteoblasts can't work properly without sufficient osteoclast activity. Each year, our bodies replace about 5-10% of all our bone tissue in this way, so let's take a closer look at this process.

Since osteoclasts (from the Greek roots *osteo* for bone and *klast* for break) originate in the immune system, bone formation requires an optimally functioning immune system. Osteoclasts break down the protein, calcium, phosphorous, and other minerals in bone and release them back into the blood stream. Osteoblasts (*blast* is another Greek root meaning sprout) come along behind and construct bone matrix, filling it with calcium. They also secrete collagen and gly-coproteins onto the surface of the bone in order for proper mineral-ization to occur. The osteoblast then imbeds itself into the bone and becomes an osteocyte (bone cell), thereby building and maintaining the new bone in the process called deposition, mineralization, or remodeling.

Other Factors Associated with Bone Building

Other factors besides osteoclasts and osteoblasts regulate bone resorption and mineralization, including hormones, nutrients, and cytokines, which are chemicals produced by the immune system. Since both cytokines and osteoclasts are produced by the immune system, you can see how vital your immune system is to bone health. Here's yet another immune system connection. During periods of inflammation or infection, your immune system produces nitric oxide, which can cause excessive bone resorption. On the other hand, normal levels of nitric oxide prevent bone resorption.

Another substance to watch out for is homocysteine, which is a pro-inflammatory blood acid linked to other inflammatory con-ditions like heart attack, stroke, and Alzheimer's disease. A recent report published in the *New England Journal of Medicine* indicates that high levels of homocysteine inhibit new bone formation by interrupting the cross-linking of collagen fibers in bone tissue, and new studies are showing that high levels of homocysteine double the risk of osteoporosis-related fractures. Another reason you don't want high levels of homocysteine is that your body likes to keep your blood slightly alkaline and will pull calcium out of your bones if necessary to neutralize acidic blood. A blood test can check your level of homocysteine, vitamin B12, vitamin B6, and folic acid (another B vitamin), which all reduce homocysteine. Some people have a genetic factor that renders them incapable of converting folic acid to its active form, so if your homocysteine level remains high, even after several weeks of vitamin B supplementation, you can use a more bio-available form called 5-methyl-tetrahydrofolate.

Normal Bone Loss and Osteoporosis

In most women, bone mass peaks between the ages of twenty and thirty, but the timing can vary somewhat, depending on race and lifestyle. It is normal to lose some bone with age, so at some point in your mid-to-late thirties, bone resorption will begin to outpace bone formation. Starting at that time, it's normal to lose 0.5-1.0% of bone mass per year until menopause. Thereafter, during the peri-menopausal/menopausal years, the rate normally accelerates to 1.0-5.0% per year because of the dip in reproductive hormones. Within five years after menopause, once hormonal fluctuation settles down, bone loss evens out again to a gradual and perfectly normal decline of 1.0-1.5% per year.

The Effect of Hormones on the Bone Building Process

All of the sex hormones play a critical role in this complex process of bone breakdown and formation; this connection is so strong that the rate of bone resorption and formation fluctuates with the menstrual cycle. Bone resorption (removal of old bone) occurs primarily during the follicular phase of the cycle (approximately Days 1-14) when estrogen is the dominant hormone. Bone remodeling takes place during the luteal phase of the menstrual cycle, (approximately Days 15-28) when progesterone is the dominant hormone.

Progesterone

It's no coincidence that the process of bone loss normally begins in the mid-thirties, just when progesterone production begins to wane. The reason for the correlation is that progesterone facilitates osteo-blastic (bone-building) activity. In fact, progesterone is essential for the synthesis of osteoblasts, and we now know that osteoblasts contain progesterone receptors, demonstrating the need for progesterone to attach to them. So, it's not surprising that John Lee, M.D., author of several books on progesterone, found that his patients' bone density increased 7-8% in the first year of progesterone use (20 mg of progesterone twice daily). This finding is extremely amazing. Let's just bear in mind that his patients had normal levels of estrogen or were taking estrogen too. His study is just one related to progesterone's ability to increase bone density as reviewed in chapter 3.

Estrogen

We know that menopause results from a drop in estrogen, and since estrogen subdues (or slows down) the osteoclasts that remove bone cells, it's not surprising that bone loss accelerates to an average of 2-3% per year immediately following menopause. While the removal (resorption) of old bone is necessary for the formation of new bone, a sharp decline in estrogen, such as the drop that often accompanies menopause, causes osteoclasts to become too aggressive, removing too much old bone before new bone can form in its place. In addition, estrogen deficiency increases the sensitivity of your bones to parathyroid hormone (PTH) (see Parathyroid Hormone section), which also increases resorption of calcium from the bones. You can see why it's so important to deal with estrogen deficiency. Estrogen directs absorption of calcium into bones and stimulates calcitonin.

Testosterone

Testosterone's anabolic (tissue-building) properties make it vitally important to the formation of bone. Testosterone increases production of osteoblasts, so it's no wonder that research has found that low testosterone levels correlate with bone loss.

Dehydroepiandrosterone

Dehydroepiandrosterone (DHEA) is a steroid hormone produced by the adrenal glands. The normal, age-related decline of DHEA is associated with many degenerative changes, including lower bone mineral density. One way DHEA works is by stimulating osteoblast activity. And osteoblasts themselves may convert DHEA to estrone, an estrogen, through a reaction regulated by vitamin D3. This conversion, in turn, would affect the production of osteoclasts that slow bone loss. In addition, DHEA inhibits pro-inflammatory cytokines such as Interleukin 6, (IL-6). In excess, IL-6 can signal cellular destruction, resulting in bone loss. Unfortunately, IL-6 rises with age while DHEA declines. Interestingly, osteoblasts also secrete IL-6 to stimulate osteoclast formation, so if osteoblast synthesis is lower than it ought to be, your body creates fewer of the osteoclasts it needs to remove old bone cells to make way for the new.

Cortisol

Another hormone that strongly affects skeletal health is cortisol. As you now know, it's normal for cortisol levels to rise in response to adrenal stressors like mental stress, physical insults, chemical exposure, and blood sugar imbalance. Acute stress is supposed to stimulate cortisol production, but persistent stressors may cause long-term exposure to high levels of cortisol. As we have noted several times, chronically elevated cortisol causes numerous problems. Excess cortisol suppresses the immune system, and its catabolic (tissue-dissolving) properties may deplete bone and block osteoblast action. Cortisol can also block calcium absorption in the intestines and deplete magnesium, thereby reducing bone formation. Of course, it's fine for all these things to occur during a short-term response to acute stress; cortisol does these things to enable you to respond quickly to a threat. It's chronically elevated cortisol that poses a threat to your bones and other parts of your body.

Melatonin

Melatonin is a hormone produced by the pineal gland in the brain. Though we associate it with sleep, it is found in abundance in bone marrow, where the bone cell precursors are, and recent studies indicate that melatonin may help prevent bone loss in several ways. It inhibits excess osteoclast formation, and therefore, excess bone resorption. It also triggers production of bone matrix proteins. Melatonin promotes the formation of osteoblasts and the production of collagen, which is necessary for bone formation. Additionally, melatonin promotes circadian secretion of human growth hormone, which promotes bone building. Unfortunately, as with so many other hormones, melatonin production declines with age.

Parathyroid Hormone

Another hormone that affects bone health is Parathyroid hormone (PTH), which is partially responsible for maintaining adequate calcium levels in your blood. When the calcium level in your blood drops below a certain point, the tiny parathyroid glands located behind the thyroid gland secrete PTH, which decreases the amount of calcium excreted by your kidneys. If necessary, it also stimulates calcium and phosphate resorption from the bones to ensure adequate blood calcium levels for normal body functions. Finally, PTH activates vitamin D and converts it to calcitriol. Calcitriol's job is to increase calcium absorption in the small intestine in order to increase blood calcium levels without withdrawing calcium from your bones. As is so often the case, PTH is beneficial to your bones in the right amount and in proper balance with other hormones. Estrogen deficiency can increase the sensitivity of bones to PTH, thereby increasing resorption. PTH is available by prescription for the treatment of both men and women at high risk of fracture. Typically injected daily, it is now available as a prescription nasal spray. The spray can cause nasal irritation, headache, and joint pain. While side effects of PTH are generally mild, high doses caused bone cancer in rats, so treatment is limited to two years.

Calcitonin

When blood calcium levels rise above a certain level, the thyroid glands secretes calcitonin, which normalizes blood calcium levels and channels excess calcium to bone formation. Calcitonin also decreases osteoclast activity to prevent excess resorption, while increasing osteoblast activity to increase mineralization. Prescription calcitonin increases bone mass in women more than five years past menopause.

Bone Health and Fractures

Bones need to be flexible as well as strong to prevent fracture under stress, and some experts believe that bone density doesn't necessarily indicate bone strength and flexibility. That is, bones can be very dense, meaning rich in calcium, and very hard, but also brittle. The key to bone health is the collagen matrix, which is a foundation of nutrients and minerals that allows bone to expand, contract, and bend without breaking. A healthy collagen matrix keeps the mineralized bone supple and resilient.

Bone-Building Nutrients

Calcium

When healthy, our bones are the storage site for about 99% of our total calcium, along with 85% of our phosphorous and 50% of our sodium and magnesium. The other 1% of our calcium performs other physiological functions, including nerve transmission, blood clotting, muscle growth and contraction, heart function, activation of enzymes, hormone function, and metabolism. Calcium also protects against colon polyps, especially the type most likely to turn cancerous. Since our bodies need calcium to function, when there's a shortage our bodies pull calcium from our bones.

Many experts believe Americans get plenty of calcium from our food. So why do so many of us have osteoporosis? Well, it's not enough to consume adequate calcium. You have to be able to absorb and use the calcium you get, so the first hurdle is digestion. You need a certain amount of stomach acid to digest calcium, and unfortunately, stomach acid production decreases with age. (Funny how antacid commercials lead you to believe that the calcium in antacids builds bones, when what it really does is prevent the absorption of the calcium you are getting.) And you need certain vitamins and minerals, especially magnesium, along with calcium in order to build bone. What many people don't realize is that if they take calcium without all the necessary co-factors, it can't be used to build bones; it can instead be deposited in joints, causing stiffening and bone spurs. Or, it can be deposited in blood vessels as plaque or in your kidneys, causing kidney stones. So if you're deficient in any key nutrients, no matter how much calcium you eat or take as a supplement, your body may not necessarily be using it to build bones.

Another factor to consider is excess calcium loss. Ingesting excess protein, sugar, caffeine, and colas will cause our bodies to excrete our valuable calcium. Problems with teeth, hair, and nails can all be signs of calcium deficiency.

We know that calcium supplementation can improve bone density in pre- and perimenopausal women. We also know that in postmenopausal women calcium supplements can slow bone loss and protect against hip fracture. Unfortunately, some women don't tolerate calcium supplements very well, experiencing constipation or bloating. One cause of this unpleasantness is taking a poorly absorbable form of calcium that blocks stomach acid production, namely the calcium carbonate found in antacids and many calcium supplements. Another cause of poor tolerance of calcium supplementation is lack of magnesium. Here's why you have to have magnesium. The intestine is a muscle that contracts in a rhythmic, wavelike motion called peristalsis to move waste through and out of the body. The intestine must be relaxed in order for peristalsis to occur. Since calcium causes muscles to tighten, while magnesium helps your muscles relax, calcium without adequate magnesium can cause your intestine to tighten, often leading to constipation. People who get constipated when they're nervous can relate.

Foods high in calcium are collards, kale, turnip greens, almonds, brazil nuts, sunflower seeds, olives, sesame seeds, and walnuts. Note that calcium from dairy products is not necessarily absorbed very well and can worsen allergies and sinus congestion.

There are two things to consider when purchasing calcium supplements. First, many forms of calcium are available, some of which are much more easily absorbed than others. The most absorbable forms are hydroxyapatite, citrate, malate, bisglycinate and chelate. The least absorbable forms are milk calcium and calcium carbonate. Second, don't buy plain calcium without the necessary co-factors that enable your body to use calcium. Many companies now promote food based calcium supplements as being superior.
Recommended amount: 1000-1500 mg in divided doses daily

Boron

Boron is a trace mineral essential to healthy bone and joint function. Research indicates an association between boron deficiency and higher risk of postmenopausal bone loss. Boron is necessary for the activation of vitamin D, which in turn stimulates absorption and utilization of calcium; it also reduces excretion of calcium, magnesium, vitamin D, and potassium. It has even been demonstrated to increase blood-serum concentrations of estrogen and testosterone, both of which are essential to bone-building and the prevention of bone loss.
Recommended amount: 1-3 mg daily.

Vitamin D

Vitamin D performs both hormonal and nutritional functions. In its active, hormonal form, vitamin D works with stomach acid and other vitamins to enhance absorption of calcium from the small intestine into the bloodstream. It also allows the kidneys to reabsorb calcium that might otherwise be excreted. Vitamin D deficiency results in inadequate skeletal mineralization (rickets in children) or mineral depletion (osteomalacia in adults). When a vitamin D deficiency exists, PTH production increases to compensate for the calcium deficiency, with the unfortunate result of excess bone resorption. One research study showed that up to 30-40% of older patients with hip fractures had vitamin D deficiencies. Whether ingested or created naturally by the action of sunlight on the skin, vitamin D3 is carried to internal organs, where it is converted to its potent hormonal form.

Please ask your physician to check your vitamin D level. Even though the lab range for normal vitamin D levels is 32 to 100, an optimal level should be 60 to 80. Before you start taking vitamin D, make sure it is vitamin D3 instead of vitamin D2, the synthetic form. This web site has some very helpful information about vitamin D: http://vitamindcouncil.org/
Recommended amount: 2000-4000 or more IU daily.

Silicon/Silica

Silicon appears to be essential for proper functioning of an enzyme that assists with the formation of collagen in bone, cartilage, and connective tissues, and it may also play a role in bone calcification. We know that silicon deficiency causes bone defects in animals, and in a small human study, women who took silica showed significantly increased bone mineral density in the femur (thighbone). Traditional herbal medicine recommends a silicon-rich plant called horsetail to heal and build bones.

Vitamin K

By slowing calcium loss and increasing levels of the bone-building protein gamma carboxyglutamic acid, vitamin K ensures that calcium goes into the bones and stays out of areas of the body, like the arteries, where it does not belong. Vitamin K is also essential for activation of osteocalcin, a substance found in the non-collagenous protein in bone and believed to play a role in bone formation.

Because vitamin K is involved in blood clotting and may interact with certain medications, you should not take it if you are taking anti-coagulant drugs like Coumadin®.
Recommended amount: 100 mcg daily.

Vitamin C

Vitamin C is essential for the formation of collagen, the primary structural protein component in bone. This is why bones break so easily and tissues are so weak in people with scurvy, the overt form of Vitamin C deficiency.

Recommendations vary widely: 500 to 3,000 mg daily in divided doses.

Flaxseed

Flaxseed has been shown to significantly reduce the rate of bone loss in postmenopausal women with thinning bones.

Recommended amount: 2-4 tablespoons of ground flaxseed sprinkled on foods or blended into a smoothie.

Fish Oil

Fish oil protects against bone loss by curbing overzealous osteoclast activity and therefore excess bone resorption. The omega-3 fatty acids in fish oil may temper the activity of pro-inflammatory cytokines, which play a major role in a variety of immunological, inflammatory, and infectious diseases.

Recommendations range from 1200 mg to 4000 mg daily.

Zinc

Zinc is necessary for bone formation, and zinc deficiency is associated with decreased bone density.

Recommended amount: 15 mg or more daily.

Magnesium

As necessary as calcium is for increasing bone density, magnesium is involved in a number of activities supporting bone strength, preservation, and remodeling. It strongly affects osteoblast and osteoclast activity and increases calcium absorption from the blood into the bone. As mentioned earlier, magnesium causes muscles to relax while calcium causes muscles to contract, making a proper balance between calcium and magnesium necessary to keep your heart muscle working properly. Because excess calcium can cause excessive contractions in the heart, doctors sometimes prescribe calcium channel blockers to prevent excess calcium from causing excessive heart contractions. Magnesium is a natural calcium channel blocker, and several research studies suggest that the vast majority of heart attack sufferers have magnesium deficiencies.

As an added bonus, magnesium has been demonstrated to help with migraines, insomnia, depression, PMS, high blood pressure, backache, constipation, kidney stones, chronic fatigue, insulin resistance, and chocolate cravings. So remember, no amount of calcium you consume can improve your bones without adequate magnesium. Magnesium deficiency is very common in the U.S. because many people don't eat enough magnesium-rich dark green leafy vegetables. Dairy products contain little magnesium, and ironically, too much calcium can block magnesium absorption. Alcohol also depletes magnesium stores. Some of the symptoms of magnesium deficiency are hair loss, muscle cramps, irritability, trembling, and disorientation. Better forms of magnesium are citrate, chelate, glycinate, and lactate, while magnesium oxide is considered to be less absorbable.

Recommended amount: 400 mg or more daily.

Manganese

Manganese plays a role in the deposition of calcium into the bones.

Recommended amount: 1 mg daily.

Phosphorus

Phosphorus is necessary for the proper utilization of calcium and for bone formation. A good balance between calcium and phosphorous (about 5:1) is vital to bone strength, but many American women are phosphorus-deficient, especially since phosphorus

deficiency increases with age. On the other hand, excess phosphorus depletes calcium.
Recommended amount: 500 mg daily.

Folic Acid, B6, and B12

Since elevated homocysteine interferes with the formation of collagen, it's not surprising that research shows that it doubles the risk of osteoporosis-related fractures. Excess homocysteine also increases the risk of cardiovascular disease. Fortunately, vitamins B6, B12 and folic acid help reduce homocysteine.
Recommended amounts:
Folic acid: 400 to 800 mcg daily.
B6: 25 mg or more daily.
B12: 500-2000 mcg.

Strontium

A fairly new discovery is that the trace mineral strontium is important to bone health. In fact, it appears to be one of the most effective substances yet discovered for preventing and treating osteoporosis. Because its molecular structure is similar to that of calcium, strontium is incorporated onto the crystal surface of bone. It can replace lost calcium in the bones and teeth and increase bone density. A research paper in the *New England Journal of Medicine* reported results of a three-year study of 1649 women with osteoporosis who took 1000 mg of strontium daily. These women showed statistically significant increases in bone mineral density of the hip, thigh (8.3%), and lumbar spine (14%), and the incidence of hip fracture dropped by 49% the first year. The number of vertebral fractures decreased as well. The levels of biochemical markers for bone resorption indicated that the rate of bone resorption did not change, leading researchers to conclude that one thousand milligrams daily of strontium increased bone formation without increasing bone resorption, that is removal of old bone. Maybe the most amazing finding was the lack of side effects; those taking the placebo actually reported more side effects than those taking strontium. Research participants also took calcium and vitamin D supplements to normalize their blood levels of these nutrients.

In rats, strontium was shown to reverse bone loss induced by estrogen deficiency, and another recent study demonstrated that taking strontium for slightly over six months improved bone mineral density for years afterward. Strontium is now available by prescription in Europe as a medication Protelos® (a salt of strontium and ranelic acid). In fact, Protelos® is the first dual-action osteoporosis drug on the market, increasing new bone formation while decreasing resorption. In other words, it slows the removal of old bone and increases bone building. Two large multi-national research studies have demonstrated the safety and effectiveness of Protelos® at a dose of 200 mg daily. One of these studies, called The Spinal Osteoporosis Therapeutic Intervention trial, found that Protelos® reduced the risk of a new vertebral fracture by 41% after three years, compared with placebo. The Treatment of Peripheral Osteoporosis study found a 16% reduction in non-vertebral fractures in all patients and a 36% reduction in hip fractures among high-risk patients. In both studies, Protelos® was well tolerated with fewer side effects than existing osteoporosis drugs. But you don't even need a prescription to take advantage of strontium's benefits because strontium citrate is available without a prescription. Let me give one cautionary note, though; animal research suggests that if you're calcium deficient increasing dietary intake of strontium may actually demineralize your bones, so be sure that along with strontium you get plenty of calcium (in an easily absorbable form) and vitamin D. Take Strontium at a different time of day than you take your calcium supplement. People on kidney dialysis should not use strontium supplements.

Recommended amount: 800 to 1000 mg a day of strontium citrate.

Ipriflavone

A derivative of a plant compound called isoflavone, ipriflavone is already used in several countries as a prescription medication for prevention and treatment of osteoporosis. Sixty clinical studies around the world have found that ipriflavone inhibits bone resorption while increasing formation of new bone. Research also shows that ipriflavone increases bone formation in both men and women. It has been shown to increase bone density, reduce the incidence of vertebral fractures, significantly reduce bone pain, and improve mobility in postmenopausal women suffering from bone loss. Ipriflavone also enhances calcitonin's effects on calcium metabolism and reduces biological markers for bone breakdown by 29%. Some research has even found that ipriflavone increased bone density by 2% in six months and 5.8% by twelve months. Studies have also demonstrated that long-term treatment with ipriflavone can be considered safe. Caution: always use a good, easily absorbable calcium supplement along with ipriflavone.

Recommended amount: 600 mg daily in divided doses.

Prescription Medications for Osteopenia and Osteoporosis

Biphosphonates

Biphosphonates are a class of drugs frequently prescribed for osteoporosis, including alendronate (Fosamax), ibandronate (Boniva), and risedronate (Actonel). Bisphosphonates are prescription drugs that interfere with osteoclast function and reduce the number of osteoclasts. You may not know that these chemicals were originally used in industrial corrosion prevention, laundry soaps, and fertilizer. In the late 1960s, researchers found that Bisphosphonates inhibit bone resorption. After osteopenia was classified as a medical condition in 1994, the Food and Drug Administration (FDA) approved Fosamax in 1995 for the treatment and prevention of osteoporosis. Sales are now in the billions of dollars a year.

How They Work

Fosamax works by inhibiting bone resorption, which sounds helpful. However, as we've learned, bone remodeling is a two-part process. If resorption is delayed, so is formation. True, bisphosphonates prevent bone loss, but they do not stimulate new bone building, and while the bone may appear to be more dense, it is old and brittle. None of the studies suggest that these medications increase bone flexibility.

Questionable Results

Women taking Fosamax showed a 4.6% increase in bone density, while Actonel improved bone density by only 2.5%. These increases are small, and within the 3-5% margin of error for any research study. Compared with results with ipriflavone (2-6%) and strontium (8-14%), they aren't too impressive. Worse, there might be other problems with these medications.

Potential Problems

There have been no long-term research studies on the effects on bone health and overall health of patients using these drugs. During the longest study, which spanned ten years, half the test subjects dropped out, citing negative side effects and/or difficulty in following the treatment protocol. Because these medications can cause inflammation of the esophagus and stomach lining if you lie down too soon after taking them, the manufacturer directs that it be taken with a full glass of water upon rising, at least 30-60 minutes before breakfast, during which time the patient must remain upright to minimize unpleasant side effects. The manufacturer claims that the drug is safe when these precautions are followed, and some women seem to tolerate these medications just fine. However, others complain of debilitating indigestion and stomach pain. Also, some women taking Fosamax for long periods report serious bone and joint pain and decreased mobility. Other side effects are esophagitis, gastritis and diarrhea.

Several researchers have cautioned doctors and patients about using bisphosphonates in concert with some other drugs. Authors of a small research study concluded that patients shouldn't take Fosamax and naproxen (a popular NSAID; non-steroidal anti-inflammatory drug prescribed for arthritis pain) together because the drugs had a synergistic effect that promoted gastric ulcers and serious side effects.

In 1993 another research study found that 33% of the study group complained of blurred vision, and a small percentage of bisphosphonates users experienced serious eye problems that could lead to vision loss, including acute glaucoma. And one in twelve people who took corticosteroids in conjunction with bisphosphonates in a recent small study experienced bone death (osteonecrosis) in their jaws. For this reason, the American Dental Association advised dentists to insist that all patients taking these osteoporosis drugs sign a release form before undergoing invasive procedures like tooth extractions, root canals, and sometimes even fillings.

More About:

Possible adverse side effects associated with bisphosphonates

- *Ulcers of the esophagus*
- *Upper GI irritation*
- *Irregular heartbeat*
- *Fractures of the femur*
- *Low calcium in the blood*
- *Skin rash*
- *Joint, bone, and muscle pain*
- *Jaw bone decay (osteonecrosis) (rare)*
- *Increased parathyroid hormone (PTH)*

A very small study published in *The Journal of Clinical Endocrinology and Metabolism* in 2005 suggested that bisphosphonates might possibly worsen the very problems they're trying to cure. I should emphasize, though, this study does not prove that Fosamax caused the problems. This study described nine patients taking Fosamax for osteopenia or osteoporosis who experienced non-traumatic fractures, that is, fractures that occur without force being applied to the bone. Six of these women experienced delayed or no healing of the broken bones while they were still taking the bisphosphonates. One osteoporotic woman's thighbone broke when she was jolted on the subway. It took two years to heal, and the healing occurred only after she stopped taking Fosamax. A year later, after she started taking Fosamax again, she broke her foot.

We are told that the benefits of bisphosphonates outweigh the risks, but in my opinion, there are more effective ways to rebuild bone without the risks.

Raloxifene (Evista®)

Evista, another medication often prescribed for bone loss, is one of a class of drugs called *selective estrogen receptor modulators*, or SERMs for short. SERMs selectively bind to the estrogen receptor sites in osteoclasts, slowing bone loss. I say selectively because, while SERMs act like estrogen in osteoclasts, they do not have similar effects in other estrogen-sensitive tissue such as that in the breast or uterus. The action of SERMs in osteoclasts decreases the rate of bone turnover in postmenopausal women, but remember that decreasing bone loss is only half of the equation. Side effects include increased hot flashes, leg cramps, flu-like symptoms, blood clots, and peripheral edema. People with liver disease should not take Evista. Oddly enough, little is seen or heard about the manufacturer's pre-market clearance study, which showed that Evista induced ovarian cancer in mice and rats. Alarmingly, the researchers saw carcinogenic effects at dosages well below the recommended therapeutic level.

Since Raloxifene (Evista) is related to tamoxifen (Nolvadex®), which has been used for many years in breast cancer patients, researchers conducted a study to determine whether Evista would offer women a clearly safer alternative to tamoxifen for breast cancer prevention. Hopes were dashed when the long-awaited results were published in 2006. The post-menopausal women in the trial all had risk factors for coronary heart disease and were considered at risk for heart attack and stroke. Though the women who took Evista did develop significantly fewer breast cancers in the approximately five-year study, they also had significantly more fatal strokes and potentially dangerous blood clots. Therefore, researchers concluded that the benefits of Evista for preventing osteoporosis and breast cancer have to be weighed against the risk of stroke and blood clots on a case-by-case basis.

Summary

I would like to make a few comments about osteoporosis, osteopenia, testing, and treatment. Women of all ages should make sure that they get adequate levels of all bone-building nutrients throughout their lives. You should also have a DEXA test. If the results show osteopenia or osteoporosis, don't panic; bone loss can be reversed. The first step is to have your estrogen, progesterone, testosterone, DHEA, and cortisol checked. Based on the test results, take the bioidentical hormones indicated and nutritional supplementation necessary to bring hormone levels into the normal ranges. Then take bone-building nutrients, remembering that most multi-vitamins don't contain adequate levels of these key nutrients. Since obviously you can't take all these nutrients individually, look for bone-building supplements that include as many of these nutrients as possible. Purchase the best bone-building formula you can find, and be prepared to pay more than you would expect because sometimes the more absorbable forms of these nutrients are more expensive. Remember, in this case, quality is everything. In addition, if you have lost bone, consider taking strontium or ipriflavone. Educate yourself on weight-bearing exercises, and start an exercise program approved by your doctor to enhance bone building. After you've done all that, you're going to need to be patient because it takes time for your body to build bone—maybe even a year or more. Get tested again after a year. If no further bone loss has occurred, rejoice! That is good news. Once your bones stop losing mass, density should start increasing. I've seen it happen many times, and it can happen for you as well.

CONCLUSION

STEP 7: LOVE YOURSELF ENOUGH TO INVEST IN YOU

The power of a hormone makeover can truly affect every area of your life. It is important. You are important. The details and responsibilities of your life are important. Don't set aside this information, and don't set aside caring for yourself. Women are often guilty of not taking care of themselves while they bend over backwards to take care of everyone else. A hormone makeover will require sacrifice of time and money. Treatment, hormones, and supplements cost money. It really is okay to spend some time and money on yourself. It does not mean that you are depriving others to do so. Investing in your health means improved quality of life, not only for you but also for those precious loved ones too. It could mean you have more energy to spend with them and do what you need to do. It could mean you feel calmer or more motivated. It could mean that you are preventing age-related diseases so your family members won't have to take care of you down the road. Sacrificing your health does not benefit your family. Bless yourself and your loved ones by investing in yourself. Get started on your hormone makeover today. You deserve it!

Don't let fear, confusion, or even ridicule from medical professionals prevent you from achieving hormone balance. To those who think there is no research on BHRT, you are wrong. I have the extensive listing of medical studies with supporting evidence regarding

BHRT in the back of this book. In fact one third of this entire book is just that—actual studies. Yes, there is more than ample medical research to support the use of BHRT and supplementation. The references are printed in the next chapter. If this is all new to your physician, he or she can even work with you through the services at www.donnawhitehormonemakeover.com. So now what, once you have experienced a fantastic hormone makeover? My hope is that you do two things: fulfill your God-given destiny with energy and renewed passion and then tell another woman about this book. Your sisters, friends, and colleagues deserve to have the life changing benefits of balanced hormones too.

With all of my heart, I hope this book is a blessing to you.
Donna

GLOSSARY

Glossary provided compliments of ZRT Laboratory in Beaverton, OR. www.zrtlab.com

ADRENAL GLANDS - produce several hormones including cortisol and DHEA. These glands take over at menopause to become the main source of all hormone production in the body.

ADRENAL IMBALANCE - also known as low adrenal reserve or adrenal insufficiency, leading to adrenal fatigue. This condition occurs when the adrenals no longer produce enough hormones to meet bodily demand and is a result of prolonged stress (emotional, viral, physical). Adrenal support includes adequate rest, exercise, nutrition, and supplementation with physician guidance.

ADRENOCORTICOTROPIN (ACTH) - hormone made by the pituitary gland that stimulates production of adrenal hormones.

ANDROGENS - testosterone and DHEA (anabolic hormones) that build and maintain skin, bone, and muscle. DHEA, the principal androgen in both men and women, is linked to energy, immune function, mood, and mental function. Testosterone is necessary to maintain muscle mass, bone density, skin elasticity, sex drive, and cardiovascular health in both sexes.

ANDROGEN DOMINANCE - excessive androgens, relative to inadequate estrogen or progesterone levels, that are produced endogenously (within the body) or with supplementation can lead to symptoms of acne, increased facial/body hair, and loss of scalp hair.

ANDROPAUSE - also called male menopause. Occurs as male hormones, testosterone and DHEA, decrease with age.

ANDROSTENEDIONE - an androgen that is necessary for the synthesis of both estrogen and testosterone.

ANOVULATION/ANOVULATORY - suspension or cessation of ovulation.

AROMATASE - an enzyme found predominantly in fat tissue that converts androgens to estrogens.

BIOAVAILABLE - the unbound (free) fraction of a hormone that has left the bloodstream to enter target tissues in the body. This unbound fraction is present and measurable in saliva.

BIOIDENTICAL - hormones derived from natural plant compounds (e.g., soy) and synthesized to duplicate the exact structure and function of hormones produced naturally within the body.

BLOOD SPOT TESTING - a minimally invasive technique for testing hormones and other substances using drops of blood that are dried on special filter paper. Blood spot testing avoids the discomfort and inconvenience of having blood drawn at the doctor's office, and simple finger or heel stick reduces pain and stress that can alter accuracy of results.

COMPOUNDING PHARMACIST - a pharmacist skilled in formulating natural, bioidentical hormone supplements based on tested hormone levels and tailored to individual patient needs.

CORPUS LUTEUM - formed from the ruptured ovarian follicle that released the egg; it produces progesterone.

CORTISOL - produced by the adrenal glands, this hormone regulates the stress response, glucose metabolism, and immune function. Cortisol has a catabolic (breaking down) action on tissue when levels are too high or out of balance, leading to low immunities, allergies, and stress-related illness.

DHEA (DEHYDROEPIANDROSTERONE) - hormone produced primarily by the adrenal glands that converts to androgens and estrogens. Its actions influence energy, stamina, mental outlook, and immune function.

DIHYDROTESTOSTERONE (DHT) - a biologically active metabolite of the hormone, testosterone, formed primarily in the prostate gland, testes, hair follicles, and adrenal glands by the enzyme 5α-reductase. DHT is three times more potent than testosterone. It is associated with male pattern baldness and prostate problems, is crucial to virilization (male gender differentiation), and reduces estrogen's negative effects in men.

ENDOCRINE SYSTEM - the group of glands that produce the majority of the body's hormones.

DOWN-REGULATION OF RECEPTOR SITES - a negative feedback cycle, due to excess hormone levels, that results in tissue desensitization and loss of cellular receptor sites wherever hormones bind to cells.

ENDOGENOUS - naturally occurring or originating within the body.

ENDOMETRIOSIS - the abnormal growth of uterine tissue (endometrium) in places outside the uterus such as on the ovaries and other pelvic structures. Associated with estrogen dominance.

ESTRADIOL - the primary and most-potent form of estrogen produced by the body during reproductive years.

ESTRIOL - the weakest, most benign of the three types of estrogen produced by the body. Thought to be protective.

ESTROGENS - a family of hormones (estradiol, estrone, estriol) that are necessary for cellular growth, differentiation of secondary sexual characteristics, and maintaining the health of the reproductive tissues, breasts, bones, skin, and the brain.

ESTROGEN DOMINANCE - an excess of estrogen in the absence of adequate levels of progesterone in women (or testosterone in men). It can result from estrogen replacement therapy, menopause, hysterectomy, birth control pills, and/or a decline in ovarian progesterone production. In men, it can result from reduced testosterone production by the testes. In either gender, it can result from exposure to pollutants and toxins (xenoestrogens). The constellation of symptoms ranges from breast tenderness and bloating, to mood swings and depression. Excess estrogens are a risk factor for the development of breast and prostrate cancers.

ESTRONE - one of the three types of estrogen produced by the body.

FIBROCYSTIC BREASTS - tender, painful, swollen breasts; a sign of estrogen dominance.

FOLLICULAR PHASE - the first half of the menstrual cycle when estrogens build up to trigger ovulation.

FOLLICLE STIMULATING HORMONE (FSH) - pituitary hormone involved in triggering ovulation; elevated levels may mark the onset of menopause or andropause.

FREE TESTOSTERONE INDEX - ratio between the amount of testosterone and SHBG (the protein that binds up available testosterone). Indicates the amount of bioavailable, free testosterone.

FREE TRIIODOTHYRONINE (fT3) - the active form of thyroid hormone. Normal levels keep the body functioning properly and are crucial for maintenance of physical and mental health.

FREE THYROXINE (fT4) - the main (inactive) thyroid hormone. A well-regulated process causes thyroxine to generate the much more potent thyroid hormone T3 (Triiodothyronine).

FSH - see follicle stimulating hormone

GLUCOCORTIOCOIDS - hormones, primarily cortisol, produced by the adrenal glands.

GOITER - enlargement of the thyroid gland; often visible as a swelling in the neck.

HORMONE - A chemical messenger that travels through the blood-stream to regulate various body functions. Produced in glands and organs of the body and activated in cell receptor sites.

HORMONE IMBALANCE - a problem stemming from the deficiency or overproduction of one or more hormones, particularly in relationship to the other hormones with which they interact.

HYPERTHYROIDISM - overactive thyroid function. Less common than hypothyroidism.

HYPOADRENIA - low adrenal function.

HYPOTHYROIDISM - low thyroid function, often associated with hormonal imbalance (particularly estrogen dominance) and linked with cold body temperature (feeling cold all the time), weight gain, inability to lose weight, thinning hair, low libido, and depression. Women are at greatest risk, developing thyroid problems seven times more often than men, particularly during years prior to menopause.

HYSTERECTOMY - surgical removal of the uterus, which often includes the ovaries (oophorectomy). The resulting total depletion of reproductive hormones causes women to go into "surgical menopause" overnight.

INFERTILITY - the inability to become pregnant. Hormonal imbalances are a cause of infertility.

IGF-1 - see insulin-like growth factor.

INSULIN - hormone secreted by the pancreas. It "unlocks" the cells to allow glucose (sugar) from food to enter and be converted into energy.

INSULIN-LIKE GROWTH FACTOR (IGF-1 or Somatomedin C) - the most reliable indicator of human growth hormone levels. Low levels indicate Adult Growth Hormone Deficiency associated with premature aging, decreased muscle and bone mass, slowing cognitive ability, low libido, and overall reduced quality of life.

INSULIN RESISTANCE - a term used to describe the failure of the tissues to respond (resistance) to insulin and absorb glucose for energy production. Associated with hormonal imbalance (particularly high triglycerides, polycystic ovaries, and excess androgens). Insulin resistance leads to increased risk of cardiovascular disease, diabetes and cancer.

LH - see luteinizing hormone.

LUTEINIZING HORMONE (LH) - pituitary hormone that signals the ovaries to release an egg and to make progesterone. In men, it signals the testes to produce testosterone.

LUTEAL PHASE - the latter half of the menstrual cycle when progesterone production is at its peak.

LUTEAL INSUFFICIENCY - failure of the corpus luteum to produce adequate amounts of progesterone upon ovulation; often caused by anovulation.

MALE MENOPAUSE - see andropause.

MENSTRUATION - monthly shedding and discharge of the uterine lining and blood from the uterus as part of the reproductive cycle.

MENOPAUSE/POSTMENOPAUSE - the end of menstrual cycles; cessation of menses for 12 consecutive months. Marked by physiological decline of reproductive hormones.

OSTEOPOROSIS - bone loss influenced by low estrogen, progesterone, androgens, and/or high cortisol.

OSTEOBLASTS - bone building cells.

OSTEOCLASTS - bone destroying/reabsorbing cells.

OVARIES - egg-producing female reproductive organs that are primary sources of the female reproductive hormones, estrogen and progesterone.

OVARIAN STROMA - the inner ovarian layer that can manufacture excess testosterone with hormonal imbalance.

PANCREAS - large gland in the abdomen that secretes insulin.

PCOS - see polycystic ovarian syndrome.

PERIMENOPAUSE - the 5 to 10 years approaching menopause when reproductive hormones fluctuate as ovarian functions decline.

PHYTOESTROGENS - plant compounds (e.g. soy, black cohosh) with mild estrogen-like activity; are used as natural alternatives to relieve menopausal symptoms.

PITUITARY GLAND - pea-sized gland in the brain that produces several types of hormones that trigger and regulate the steroid hormones. (See FSH, LH.)

PMS - see premenstrual syndrome.

POLYCYSTIC OVARIAN SYNDROME (PCOS) - a condition whereby undeveloped follicles (cysts) form within the ovaries. It is seen in women with high estrogen and low progesterone levels, and/ or high androgen (testosterone) and insulin levels.

PREMENSTRUAL SYNDROME (PMS) - a set of physical and emotional symptoms that stem from hormonal imbalances and fluctuations during a woman's menstrual cycle.

PROGESTERONE/ESTRADIOL (Pg/E2) RATIO - indicates fundamental balance or imbalance between these two hormones.

PROGESTINS - synthetic hormones structurally similar to progesterone (e.g. Provera) but not naturally occurring in the body; they suppress normal ovarian production of progesterone and have been shown in studies to have negative side effects.

PROGESTERONE - a hormone produced by the ovaries after ovulation and in lesser amounts by the adrenal glands. A precursor to most of the steroid hormones, it has many vital functions, from maintaining pregnancy to regulating menstrual cycles. It has calming and diuretic properties, and enhances the beneficial effects of estrogens while balancing estrogen and preventing problems linked to estrogen excess. Progesterone also facilitates balance of other steroid hormones.

PROINFLAMMATORY STATE - A condition characterized by elevations in C-reactive protein (CRP), most often associated with an increased risk of developing cardiovascular disease and diabetes. Elevated CRP is commonly caused by obesity whereby excess adipose tissue produces high levels of inflammatory proteins released during immune response that may elicit higher CRP levels.

PROSTATE SPECIFIC ANTIGEN (PSA) - a protein produced by the prostate gland; high PSA is an important indicator of prostate enlargement. A normal PSA reading is prerequisite for initiating testosterone therapy in men.

PROTHROMBOTIC STATE - A condition characterized by increased plasma plasminogen activator inhibitor (PAI)-1 and fibrinogen, commonly present in persons with CardioMetabolic Syndrome. Fibrinogen, an acute-phase reactant like CRP, rises in response to high cytokines (regulatory proteins released by immune system cells that act as intercellular mediators during immune response) which occurs in a Proinflammatory State. Therefore, prothrombotic and proinflammatory states may be metabolically interconnected.

PSA - see prostate specific antigen.

RECEPTOR SITES - molecules on the surface of the body's cells that allow specific hormones to pass into the cell (via a lock-and-key effect) to perform their regulatory function.

SEX HORMONE BINDING GLOBULIN (SHBG) - a protein that binds to specific hormones in the bloodstream (e.g., testosterone and estrogen), limiting their availability to bodily tissues. It increases with age and excess estrogens.

SHBG - see sex hormone binding globulin.

SOMATOMEDIN C - see insulin-like growth factor.

TESTES - sperm-producing male reproductive organs that are the primary source of testosterone.

TESTOSTERONE - an anabolic hormone that builds and maintains bone and muscle mass, skin elasticity, sex drive, and cardiovascular health in both sexes. The dominant male hormone.

THYROID - gland that produces hormones that regulate metabolism. Imbalances lead to weight gain, cold body temperature, depression, hair loss, etc.

THYROID PEROXIDASE ANTIBODIES (TPO) - elevated with Hashimoto's (autoimmune) thyroiditis and is associated with polycystic ovaries in women.

THYROID STIMULATING HORMONE (TSH) - the pituitary hormone that signals the thyroid to produce T4 (Thyroxine), which converts to active T3 (Triiodothyronine).

TPO - see thyroid peroxidase antibodies.

TSH - see thyroid stimulating hormone.

TYPE 2 DIABETES - initially the pancreas makes too much insulin which cannot be taken up by the cells. Eventually the pancreas no longer makes enough insulin to process food intake and regulate blood sugar levels. It is the most common form of preventable diabetes.

TISSUE DESENSITIZATION - the inability of cells to utilize (take up) hormones.

UTERINE FIBROID - benign tumor of the uterus, often associated with hormonal imbalance.

VASOMOTOR SYMPTOMS - hot flashes/night sweats commonly begin in perimenopause; stem from hormone fluctuations which impact centers in the brain that regulate capillary dilation and perspiration.

VITAMIN D - a group of fat-soluble prohormones (hormone precursors), the two major forms of which include Vitamin D2 and Vitamin D3. Vitamin D2 (ergocalciferol) is not found in animals, but is manufactured commercially by irradiating ergosterol (a component of fungal cell membranes) with ultraviolet light. It is the predominant form for prescription use in the US, especially in high-dose preparations. Vitamin D3 (cholecalciferol), which is the natural-occuring form of Vitamin D, is produced from the reaction of ultraviolet light on the skin. This form also found in cod liver oil and Vitamin D supplements that state "cholecalciferol" in their ingredients. Vitamin D has been found to be important in protecting the body from a wide range of diseases including cardiovascular disease, stroke, osteoporosis, osteomalacia, cancer, autoimmune diseases (such as multiple sclerosis), rheumatoid arthritis, diabetes (Types 1 and 2), and schizophrenia.

REFERENCES

Commentary on studies notated with an * are from Women in Balance, a non-profit advocacy for women's hormone balance web site. http://www.womeninbalance.org/resources_and_research/

INTRODUCTION

Writing Group for the Women's Health Initiative Investigators, "Risk and benefits of estrogen plus progestin in healthy post-menopausal women," *JAMA* 2002; 288:321-333.

Grady D, Herrington D, Bittner V, et al. Cardiovascular disease outcomes during 6.8 years of hormone therapy: Heart and Estrogen/progestin Replacement Study follow-up (HERS II). *JAMA* 2002; 288(1):49-57.

CHAPTER 2

Wilson, Robert. *Feminine Forever.* Pocket Books, 1968.

Zimmerman, C. Who can we trust if FDA puts stamp on snake oil? *The Daily News;* November 8, 2009. www.wjla.com/news/stories/ 0406/321139.html. Accessed May 19, 2006. S*ales of Prempro® and Premphase®, which combine estrogen and progestin, and Premarin®, an estrogen-only pill, fell* *by more than 57% in just three years, from $2.07 billion in 2001 to $880 million in 2004.*

Available at: www.fda.gov/ohrms/dockets/ dockets/05p0411/05p-0411-cp00001-01-vol1.pdf. Accessed April 21, 2006.

Wyeth and its lawyers submitted a citizen's petition seeking FDA actions to counter what Wyeth calls "flagrant violations of the law by pharmacies compounding bioidentical hormone replacement therapy drugs that endanger public health."

Safety of Bio-Identical Hormones

Campagnoli C, Clavel-Chapelon F, Kaaks R, Peris C, Berrino F. Progestins and progesterone in hormone replacement therapy and the risk of breast cancer. *J Steroid Biochem* Mol Biol 2005; 96(2):95-108.

The authors discuss the non-progesterone-like effects of synthetic progestins, which can contribute to the increased risk of breast cancer when these are used as part of a combined hormone therapy regimen. In contrast, bioidentical progesterone does not increase the risk of breast cancer, consistent with experimental in vivo data that shows progesterone has no adverse effect on breast tissue. *

Chataigneau T, Zerr M, Chataigneau M, Hudlett F, Hirn C, Pernot F, Schini-Kerth VB. Chronic treatment with progesterone but not medroxyprogesterone acetate restores the endothelial control of vascular tone in the mesenteric artery of ovariectomized rats. *Menopause* 2004; 11(3):255-63.

This study helps explain the more beneficial effects on the cardiovascular system of progesterone compared with MPA because of its enhancement of the protective effects of endothelial cells on the arterial walls. *

Collins JJ, Ahlgrimm M. Hormone therapy - it's time for a second opinion. *Int J Pharm Compounding* 2008;12(7):123-127.

This paper highlights some counterarguments to an opinion piece by the American College of Obstetrics and Gynecologists, which has been widely quoted as evidence against the use of bioidentical hormones. The authors urge clinicians reading the ACOG opinion piece to ask themselves whether it really reflects clinical advances in the use of compounded and FDA-approved bioidentical hormones that have transformed the practice of hormone replacement therapy. They recommend that people read the original research, rather than quoting reviews and opinions that are not well founded in the literature. *

Curcio JJ, Wollner DA, Schmidt JW, Kim LS. Is Bio-Identical Hormone Replacement Therapy Safer than Traditional Hormone Replacement Therapy? A Critical Appraisal of Cardiovascular Risks in Menopausal Women. *Treat Endocrinol.* 2006; 5(6):367-374.

This review examines currently used bioidentical hormones used as alternatives to conventional hormone replacement therapy. The authors acknowledge that the clinical evidence shows natural progesterone to be superior to synthetic progestins, because of its more beneficial effects on lipids, the nervous system, and overall quality of life. Oral estriol has been associated with similar adverse effects to oral synthetic estrogens with respect to cardiovascular risks, but there is evidence that transdermal application of estrogens offers a safer alternative that "should be explored". The authors recommend longer term clinical trials of topical estriol to confirm its cardiovascular safety. *

Fournier A, Berrino F, Riboli E, Avenel V, Clavel-Chapelon F. Breast cancer risk in relation to different types of hormone replacement therapy in the E3N-EPIC cohort. *Int J Cancer* 2005; 114(3):448-54

Combined HRT with estrogen (either oral or transdermal) and synthetic progestins was found to carry a significantly increased risk of breast cancer compared with estrogens plus oral micronized progesterone. In fact, no increase in breast cancer risk was seen in the estrogen plus oral micronized progesterone group compared with estrogen alone. This large multicenter study therefore suggests that there is a dramatic difference between the effects of bioidentical progesterone versus synthetic progestins on breast cancer risk. *

Gillson GR, Zava DT. A perspective on HRT for women: picking up the pieces after the Women's Health Initiative trial - Part 1. *Int J Pharm Compounding* 2003; 7(4):250-6.

This article discusses some fundamental aspects of safer hormone replacement therapy that may have been overlooked in the debate surrounding bioidentical versus synthetic hormones: Oral delivery of hormones is not optimal; application of hormones to the skin (transdermal application) has many important advantages; and synthetic progestins are not acceptable as a substitute for natural progesterone. The evidence for and principles behind these factors are presented. *

Gillson GR, Zava DT. A perspective on HRT for women: picking up the pieces after the Women's Health Initiative trial - Part 2. *Int J Pharm* Compounding 2003; 7(5):330-8.

The authors review clinical evidence for the benefits of bioidentical progesterone over synthetic progestins. While both protect the uterine lining from proliferation caused by estrogens, progesterone has beneficial effects on cardiovascular health. The synergy between progesterone and estradiol, each "turning on" the other's receptors, has the added benefit of allowing the estradiol dosage to be reduced. Oral and transdermal dosing of bioidentical progesterone are discussed. *

Holtorf, K. 2009. The bioidentical hormone debate: Are bioidentical hormones (estradiol, estriol, and progesterone) safer or more efficacious than commonly used synthetic versions in hormone replacement therapy? *Postgrad. Med., 121* (1), 73–85.

This literature review presents the substantial evidence for the safety and efficacy of bioidentical hormone therapy, including estradiol, estriol, and progesterone, which shows that it presents lower risks for breast cancer and cardiovascular disease than synthetic or animal-derived hormones. Studies show that progestins have a number of negative effects on the cardiovascular system and an association with breast cancer risk that can be avoided by using bioidentical progesterone. This meta-analysis contains almost 200 citations and concluded that bioidentical hormones have a superior safety profile.*

Krapf JM, Simon JA. The role of testosterone in the management of hypoactive sexual desire disorder in postmenopausal women. *Maturitas.* 2009; 63(3):213-9.

This article reviews testosterone's role in sexual function in women. Research is going on to study the Safety and effectiveness of transdermal testosterone therapy in women with low sexual desire, sometimes called HSDD (hypoactive sexual desire disorder) if it leads to distress. The prevalence of this disorder is highest in women who are surgically menopausal, i.e., they have had both ovaries removed, which results in a sudden decline in testosterone levels that leads to a reduced desire for sex and less satisfying sex. The authors review clinical studies of transdermal testosterone therapy, both with and without estrogen, concluding that it is safe and effective in women struggling with HSDD. *

L'hermite, M., et al. 2008. Could transdermal estradiol + progesterone be a safer postmenopausal HRT? A review. *Maturitas, 60* (3–4), 185–201.

This detailed review examines the way different types of hormone replacement therapy (HRT) affect the cardiovascular system, the brain, and the risk of breast cancer. It discusses the research that shows that non-oral estrogens have more favorable cardiovascular effects, such as improved blood pressure control and lower risk of thrombosis. It discusses the benefits of using natural *progesterone rather than synthetic progestins in association with estrogens in HRT. Natural progesterone has a beneficial effect on blood vessels and the brain, and confers less or even no risk of breast cancer, compared with synthetic progestins.**

Moskowitz, D. 2006. A comprehensive review of the safety and efficacy of bioidentical hormones for the management of menopause and related health risks. *Altern. Med. Rev., 11* (3), 208–223.

This review describes the various synthetic estrogens and progestins used in hormone replacement therapy and discusses their safety in relation to natural alternatives. Natural estrogens and progesterone are being increasingly used in clinical practice and have demonstrated effectiveness in treating menopausal symptoms. They also have improved safety profiles with respect to breast cancer risk and cardiovascular effects.*

Schwartz ET, Holtorf K. Hormones in wellness and disease prevention: common practices, current state of the evidence, and questions for the future. *Prim Care* 2008; 35(4):669-705.

This review examines the role of hormones as critical components of overall wellness, and therefore the potential for disease prevention of ensuring that hormone levels are optimal. The authors outline age-related hormone deficiencies and supplementation strategies. The review covers estrogens, progesterone, testosterone, growth hormone and thyroid hormones, covering not only the effects of deficiency and the risk/benefit of supplementation, but also controversies surrounding such treatment. The diagnosis of hormone deficiency and monitoring of treatment is also discussed.*

Shantha S, Brooks-Gunn J, Locke RJ, Warren MP. Natural vaginal progesterone is associated with minimal psychological side effects: a preliminary study. *J Womens Health Gend Based Med* 2001; 10(10):991-7.

This 3 month, multicenter randomized study evaluated the psychological side effects of a vaginally applied progesterone gel in reproductive aged women treated for hypothalamic amenorrhea or premature ovarian failure. No differences were noted in psychometric measures as evaluated by the Hopkins Symptom Checklist. Natural progesterone in a vaginal gel can be an effective treatment for women requiring hormone therapy.*

Simon JA. Safety of estrogen/androgen regimens. *J Reprod Med* 2001; 46(3 Suppl):281-90.

Stephenson K, Price C, Kurdowska A, Neuenschwander P, Stephenson J, Pinson B, Stephenson D, Alfred D, Krupa A, Mahoney D, Zava D, Bevan M. Topical progesterone cream does not increase thrombotic and inflammatory factors in postmenopausal women. Presented at the 46th Annual Meeting of the American Society of Hematology, San Diego, December 4-7, 2004. *Blood* 2004; 104(11 Pt 1):414b-415b (Abstract 5318).

No change in any of the thrombotic or inflammatory markers studied (total factor VII:C, factor VIIa, factor V, fibrinogen, antithrombin, PAI-1, CRP, TNF?, and IL-6) was observed, despite significant symptomatic improvement compared to placebo, in 30 women receiving 20 mg/day progesterone cream for 4 weeks. This finding indicates a lack of potential adverse effects of progesterone on the cardiovascular system, particularly with respect to risk of coronary artery disease and stroke. The authors conclude that administration of topical progesterone cream at a daily dose of 20 mg significantly relieves menopausal symptoms in postmenopausal women without adversely altering prothrombotic potential. Since the thrombotic complications that are typically observed with conventional hormone replacement therapy, and have led to an increase in stroke, do not seem to occur with topical progesterone, this treatment should be seriously considered as an effective and safe alternative clinical therapy for women suffering from menopausal symptoms.*

Takahashi K, Okada M, Ozaki T, Kurioka H, Manabe A, Kanasaki H, Miyazaki K. Safety and efficacy of oestriol for symptoms of natural or surgically induced menopause. *Hum Reprod* 2000; 15(5):1028-36.

The authors gave 2 mg/day oral estriol for one year to 53 post-menopausal women (aged 40-62). None of the patients stopped treatment due to side effects; level of satisfaction with the treatment increased throughout the study, and averaged at 85% in naturally menopausal women and 93% in surgically menopausal women by the end of the year. Menopausal symptoms were significantly reduced. No distinctive effects on bone or lipid levels were seen. The authors suggest that estriol is a good choice of HRT to reduce symptoms in women who are not susceptible to osteoporosis or coronary artery disease.*

Wepfer ,ST. The science behind bioidentical hormone replacement therapy. *Int J Pharm Compounding* 2002; 6(2):142-6.

Differences between synthetic progestins and bioidentical progesterone in terms of their effects on breast cancer risk, estrogen dominance, and vasomotor symptoms are discussed. The review also covers the use of testosterone for postmenopausal women who have androgen deficiency because of surgically induced menopause. Androgen deficiency is also seen in women receiving estrogen replacement therapy, which reduces bioavailable testosterone because it increases levels of sex hormone binding globulin in the blood. The author concludes that bioidentical hormones are more effective and safer than the synthetic alternatives, but hopes that large trials will soon be conducted to confirm their promising effects.*

Safety of Bio-Identical Progesterone over Synthetic Progestins
General

de Ziegler D, Fanchin R. Progesterone and progestins: applications in gynecology. *Steroids* 2000; 65(10-11):671-9.

This paper reviews the use of a transvaginal progesterone gel as a viable option to other routes of application of natural progesterone (intramuscular, oral micronized), and offered it as a viable option to synthetic progestins given the low incidence of side effects noted in existing studies.*

L'Hermite M, Simoncini T, Fuller S, Genazzani AR. Could transdermal estradiol + Progesterone be a safer postmenopausal HRT? A review. *Maturitas* 2008;60(3-4):185-201.

This detailed review examines the way different types of hormone replacement therapy (HRT) affect the cardiovascular system, the brain, and the risk of breast cancer. It discusses the research that shows that non-oral estrogens have more favorable cardiovascular effects, such as improved blood pressure control and lower risk of thrombosis. It discusses the benefits of using natural Progesterone rather than synthetic progestins in association with estrogens in HRT. Natural progesterone has a beneficial effect on blood vessels and the brain, and confers less or even no risk of breast cancer, compared with synthetic progestins.*

Sitruk-Ware R. Progestogens in hormonal replacement therapy: new molecules, risks, and benefits. *Menopause* 2002; 9(1):6-15.

The classifications of various progestogens (natural and synthetic) are reviewed in terms of their risks and benefits. This review clearly elucidates the differences in the mode of action of various synthetic progestins as well as progesterone.

Safety of Bio-Identical Progesterone over Synthetic Progestins
Lipids and Cardiovascular

Adams MR, et al. Medroxyprogesterone acetate antagonizes inhibitory effects of conjugated equine estrogens on coronary artery atherosclerosis. *Arterioscler Throb Vasc Biol.* 1997; 17(1):217-221.

*Atherosclerotic plaque formation, progesterone is protective compared with MPA. Progesterone inhibits molecular initiators of atherosclerotic plaque formation, whereas this positive effect is not observed using MPA.**

Chataigneau T, Zerr M, Chataigneau M, Hudlett F, Hirn C, Pernot F, Schini-Kerth VB. Chronic treatment with Progesterone but not medroxyprogesterone acetate restores the endothelial control of vascular tone in the mesenteric artery of ovariectomized rats. *Menopause*. 2004; 11(3):255-63.

*This study helps explain the more beneficial effects on the cardiovascular system of Progesterone compared with MPA because of its enhancement of the protective effects of endothelial cells on the arterial walls.**

Curcio JJ, Wollner DA, Schmidt JW, Kim LS. Is Bio-Identical Hormone Replacement Therapy Safer than Traditional Hormone Replacement Therapy? A Critical Appraisal of Cardiovascular Risks in Menopausal Women. *Treat Endocrinol*. 2006; 5(6):367-374.

*This review examines currently used bioidentical hormones used as alternatives to conventional hormone replacement therapy. The authors acknowledge that the clinical evidence shows natural Progesterone to be superior to synthetic progestins, because of its more beneficial effects on lipids, the nervous system, and overall quality of life. Oral estriol has been associated with similar adverse effects to oral synthetic estrogens with respect to cardiovascular risks, but there is evidence that transdermal application of estrogens offers a safer alternative that "should be explored". The authors recommend longer term clinical trials of topical estriol to confirm its cardiovascular safety.**

Miyagawa K, et al. Medroxyprogesterone interferes with ovarian steroid protection against coronary vasospasm. *Nat Med*. 1997; 3(3):324-327.

A risk factor of cardiovascular risk is coronary spasm, which increases heart attack or stroke risk. The addition of MPA to estrogen increases vasoconstriction; the addition of bioidentical progesterone protects against artery spasm.

Rosano GM, et al. Natural progesterone, but not medroxyprogesterone acetate, enhances the beneficial effect of estrogen on exercise-induced myocardial ischemia in postmenopausal women. *J Am Coll Cardiol.* 2000; 36(7):2154-2159.

*In a blinded, randomized, crossover study, postmenopausal women with coronary artery disease were treated with estradiol for 4 weeks and then received progesterone or MPA. Exercise time to myocardial ischemia was significantly increased in the progesterone group compared with the medroxyprogesterone acetate group.**

Writing Group for the PEPI Trial. Effects of estrogen or estrogen/progestin regimens on heart disease risk factors in postmenopausal women. The Postmenopausal Estrogen/Progestin Interventions (PEPI) Trial. *JAMA.* 1995; 273(3):199-208.

*MPA negates the cardioprotective effects of estrogen. This trial was the first study to examine progesterone, progestins and Conjugated Equine Estrogens.The progestin (MPA) negatively affected high-density lipoprotein levels (HDL), but bioidentical progesterone added to CEE was associated with a significantly higher HDL level, thus sparing the beneficial lipid effects provided by CEE.**

Safety of Bio-Identical Progesterone over Synthetic Progestins
Mood

Cummings JA, Brizendine L. Comparison of physical and emotional side effects of progesterone or medroxyprogesterone in early postmenopausal women. *Menopause* 2002; 9(4):253-63.

Twenty-three early postmenopausal women were randomized to either medroxyprogesterone acetate (MPA) or oral micronized progesterone combined with conjugated equine estrogens (CEE) and followed for 91 days in a sequence of treatments. None of the hormone treatments had any noticeable effect on mood. Participants using MPA experienced more breast tenderness and bleeding than those using progesterone. This study debunks the belief that progesterone depresses mood in healthy individuals.*

Shantha S, Brooks-Gunn J, Locke RJ, Warren MP. Natural vaginal progesterone is associated with minimal psychological side effects: a preliminary study. *J Womens Health Gend Based Med* 2001; 10(10):991-7.

This 3 month, multicenter randomized study evaluated the psychological side effects of a vaginally applied progesterone gel in reproductive aged women treated for hypothalamic amenorrhea or premature ovarian failure. No differences were noted in psychometric measures as evaluated by the Hopkins Symptom Checklist. Natural progesterone in a vaginal gel can be an effective treatment for women requiring hormone therapy.*

Safety of Bio-Identical Progesterone over Synthetic Progestins
Brain and CNS

Schumacher M, Guennoun R, Ghoumari A, Massaad C, Robert F, El-Etr M, Akwa Y, Rajkowski K, Baulieu EE. Novel perspectives for Progesterone in hormone replacement therapy, with special reference to the nervous system. *Endocr Rev.* 2007; 28(4):387-439.

The authors describe in detail the neuroprotective effects of Progesterone when used in postmenopausal hormone replacement therapy. They emphasize that natural progesterone has very different properties than synthetic progestins. Medroxyprogesterone acetate actually inhibits the beneficial effects of estradiol on the nervous system and also exerts damaging effects, whereas *progesterone does neither. Progesterone is known to have neuro-protective, neurotrophic, and promyelinating effects.**

Safety of Bio-Identical Progesterone over Synthetic Progestins
Symptom Control and Quality of Life

Cummings JA, Brizendine L. Comparison of physical and emotional side effects of progesterone or medroxyprogesterone in early postmenopausal women. *Menopause*. 2002; 9(4):253-263.

*The effects of switching from synthetic progestins to progesterone showed greater satisfaction, fewer side effects and improved quality of life with progesterone as compared with MPA.**

Safety of Bio-Identical Progesterone over Synthetic Progestins
PMS

Martorano JT, Ahlgrimm M, Meyers D. Differentiating between natural progesterone and synthetic progestogens: clinical implications for premenstrual syndrome management. *Compr Ther* 1993; 19(3):96-8.

*Clinical observations demonstrate that patients suffering from PMS respond to treatment with natural progesterone, whereas synthetic progestins may exacerbate the condition. The authors review the differences between natural progesterone and synthetic progestins.**

Safety of Bio-Identical Progesterone over Synthetic Progestins
Sleep

Montplaisir J, Lorrain J, Denesle R, Petit D. Sleep in menopause: differential effects of two forms of hormone replacement therapy. *Menopause* 2001; 8(1):10-16.

This randomized clinical trial compared the effects of conjugated equine estrogen (CEE) and medroxyprogesterone acetate to CEE *and oral micronized progesterone. Twenty-one postmenopausal women were studied in a sleep lab, with results demonstrating an improvement in subjective measures of menopausal symptoms and sleep in both groups. The group receiving natural progesterone had significantly improved sleep efficiency, whereas the medroxyprogesterone acetate group did not, suggesting that the former might better improve sleep in postmenopausal women. ***

Safety of Bio-Identical Progesterone over Synthetic Progestins
Breast Cancer

Fournier A, Berrino F, Clavel-Chapelon F. Unequal risks for breast cancer associated with different hormone replacement therapies: results from the E3N cohort study. *Breast Cancer Res Treat* 2008; 107(1):103-11.

*This large multicenter study in France followed 80,377 post-menopausal women for up to 12 years, and looked in particular at whether the type of progestogen used in combination with estrogen made a difference to the risk of developing breast cancer in those women who used hormone replacement therapy (HRT). The estrogen in HRT is primarily transdermal estradiol in France. Compared with those women who did not use HRT at all, women using estrogen alone had a 1.29-fold increased risk of developing breast cancer; women using estrogen plus natural Progesterone had the same risk as women using no HRT. In women using synthetic progestins in combination with estrogen, the particular progestin used made a difference to breast cancer risk; women using dydrogesterone had a 1.16-fold increased risk of breast cancer, but those using other progestins had a 1.69-fold increased risk of breast cancer, compared to women not using HRT. The authors note that dydrogesterone is the progestin most similar to natural progesterone in its chemical structure and pharmacological effects. ***

Fournier A, et al. Breast cancer risk in relation to different types of hormone replacement therapy in the E3N-EPIC cohort. *Int J Cancer.* 2005; 114(3):448-454.

A study of more than 54,000 postmenopausal women in France found that when combined with synthetic progestins, oral and transdermal bioidentical estrogen were associated with a significantly increased risk of breast cancer. Researchers found no evidence of increased risk when estrogens were combined with bioidentical progesterone.*

Plu-Bureau G, Le MG, Thalabard JC, Sitruk-Ware R, Mauvais-Jarvis P. Percutaneous progesterone use and risk of breast cancer: results from a French cohort study of premenopausal women with benign breast disease. *Cancer Detect Prev* 1999; 23(4):290-6.

This cohort study followed 1150 premenopausal French women diagnosed with benign breast disease. Topical progesterone cream, a common treatment for mastalgia in Europe, had been prescribed to 58% of the women. Follow-up accumulated 12,462 person-years. There was no association noted between progesterone cream use and breast cancer risk. Furthermore, women who had used both progesterone cream and an oral progestogen had a significant decrease in breast cancer risk (RR= 0.5) as compared to women who did not use progesterone cream. These results suggest there are no deleterious effects caused by percutaneous progesterone use in women with benign breast disease and that different types of progestogens have different effects on mammary glands.*

Wood CE, et al. Effects of estradiol with micronized progesterone or medroxyprogesterone acetate on risk markers for breast cancer in postmenopausal monkeys. *Breast Cancer Res Treat.* 2007; 101(2):125-134.

Progestins may significantly increase estrogen-stimulated breast cell proliferation and mitotic activity, while progesterone does not.*

Women on Hormones Live Longer

Ahlgrimm, M., *The HRT Solution*. 1999; New York: Avery Publishing, p. 35.

Side Effects to Prempro

http://www.wyeth.com/content/showlabeling.asp?id=133

Side Effects to Synthetic Progesterone

Adams MR; Register TC; Golden DL; Wagner JD; Williams JK Medroxyprogesterone acetate antagonizes inhibitory effects of conjugated equine estrogens on coronary artery atherosclerosis *Arterioscler Thromb Vasc Biol* 1997 Jan;17(1):217-21 (ISSN: 1079-5642.

Clarkson TB. Progestogens and cardiovascular disease. A critical review. J Reprod Med 1999 Feb;44(2 Suppl):180-4.

Goletiani NV, Keith DR, Gorsky SJ. Progesterone: review of safety for clinical studies. *Exp Clin Psychopharmacol.* Oct; 15, 2007: (5):427-44.

Risk of venous thromboembolism is increased with estrogens plus progestins.

Levine RL; Chen SJ; Durand J; Chen YF; Oparil S. Medroxyprogesterone attenuates estrogen-mediated inhibition of neointima formation after balloon injury of the rat carotid artery. *Circulation* 1996 Nov 1;94(9):2221-7.

Miyagawa K; Rosch J; Stanczyk F; Hermsmeyer K. Medroxyprogesterone interferes with ovarian steroid protection against coronary vasospasm. *Nat Med* 1997 Mar;3(3):324-7.

Rachoń D, Teede H. Postmenopausal hormone therapy and the risk of venous thromboembolism. *Climacteric.* 2008 Aug; 11(4):273-9.

Sitruk-Ware R. Progestins and cardiovascular risk markers. *Steroids* 2000 Oct-Nov;65(10-11):651-8.

http://media.pfizer.com/files/products/uspi_provera.pdf

Side Effects to Conjugated Equine Estrogen

http://www.wyeth.com/content/showlabeling.asp?id=131

Shen L, et al. Alkylation of 2'-deoxynucleosides and DNA by the Premarin metabolite 4-hydroxyequilenin semiquinone radical. *Chem Res Toxicol.* 1998;11(2)94-101.

CEE metabolites could result in DNA damage, which may play a role in the carcinogenic effects of this type of estrogen.

HRT and Ovarian Cancer

Lacey JV, Mink PJ, Lubin JH, et al: Menopausal Hormone Replacement Therapy and Risk of Ovarian Cancer. *Journal of the American Medical Association,* Jul 17, 2002; 288(3):334-341.

Mørch, L., et al. 2009. Hormone therapy and ovarian cancer. *Journal of the American Medical Association, 203* (3), 298–305.

Side Effects of HRT

Anderson GL, Judd HL, Kaunitz AM, et al. Effects of estrogen plus progestin on gynecologic cancers and associated diagnostic procedures: The Women's Health Initiative randomized trial. *Journal of the American Medical Association* 2003; 290(13):1739–1748.

Canonico, M., et al. 2007. Hormone therapy and venous thrombo-embolism among postmenopausal women: Impact of the route of administration and progestogens: The ESTHER study. *Circulation, 115,* 840–845.

Chlebowski, R., et al. 2009. Breast cancer after use of estrogen plus progestin in postmenopausal women. *NEJM, 360* (6), 573–587.

Chlebowski, R., & Prentice, R. 2008. Menopausal hormone therapy in BRCA1 mutation carriers: Uncertainty and caution. *J. Natl. Cancer Inst., 100* (19), 1341–1343.

Craig, M., et al. 2005. The Women's Health Initiative Memory Study (WHIMS): Findings and implications for treatment. *Lancet Neurol., 4* (3), 190–194.

Eisen, A., et al. 2008. Hormone therapy and the risk of breast cancer in *BRCA1* mutation carriers. *J. Natl. Cancer Inst., 100* (19), 1361-1367.

Ewertz M, et al. Hommone use for menopausal symptoms and risk of breast cancer. A Danish cohort study. *Br J Cancer.* 2005;92(7):1293-1297.

Feeman WE. Thrombotic stroke in an otherwise healthy middle-aged female related to the use of continuous-combined conjugated equine estrogens and medroxyprogesterone acetate. *J Gend Specif Med* 2000 Nov-Dec;3(8):62-4; discussion 64-5.

Fox, M. 2009. Study makes stronger case HRT causes breast cancer. URL: http://uk.reuters.com/article/idUKN0430289320090204

Current use of synthetic HT increased breast cancer risk by 61% in women over 50 years of age.

Godsland, I. 2001. Effects of postmenopausal hormone replacement therapy on lipid, lipoprotein, and apolipoprotein (a) concentrations: Analysis of studies published from 1974–2000. *Fertil. Steril., 75* (5), 898–915.

Grady, D., et al. 2002. Cardiovascular disease outcomes during 6.8 years of hormone therapy: Heart and Estrogen/Progestin Replacement Study Follow-Up (HERS II). *JAMA, 288* (1), 49–57.

Grady, D., et al. 2000. Postmenopausal hormone therapy increases risk for venous thromboembolic disease: The Heart and Estrogen/ progestin Replacement Study (HERS). *Ann. Int. Med., 132* (9), 689–696.

Grant, C. 2008. Hormone replacement therapy. Irresponsible to modify current guidelines. Letters. *BMJ, 337*, a1494.

Heiss G., et al., WHI Investigators. 2008. Health risks and benefits 3 years after stopping randomized treatment with estrogen and pro-gestin. *JAMA, 299* (9), 1036–1045.

Women taking HRT faced a small increased risk for cancer for more than two years after they stopped taking the HRT medication.

Hulley, S., et al. 2002. Noncardiovascular disease outcomes during 6.8 years of hormone therapy: Heart and Estrogen/Progestin Replacement Study follow-up (HERS II). *JAMA, 288* (1), 58-64.

Koomen, E., et al. 2009. Estrogens, oral contraceptives and hor-monal replacement therapy increase the incidence of cutaneous melanoma: A population-based case-control study. *Ann. Oncol., 20* (2), 358–364.

Lee SA, et al. An overview of menopausal oestrogen-pro-gestin hormone therapy and breast cancer risk. *Br J Cancer.* 2005;92(11):2049-2058.

A meta-analysis of 61 studies documented a consistent increase in breast cancer risk with synthetic HT. The average increase was 7.6% per years of use, with higher doses conferring a significantly higher risk.

Micheletti, M–C., & Chevalier, T. 2007. Letter by Micheletti & Chevallier regarding article, "Hormone therapy and venous thromboembolism among postmenopausal women: Impact of the route of estrogen administration and progestogens: The ESTHER study." *Circulation, 116* (13), e362.

Modena, M., et al. 2005. New evidence regarding hormone replacement therapies is urgently required; transdermal postmenopausal hormone therapy differs from oral hormone therapy in risks and benefits. *Maturitas, 52* (1), 1–10.

Resnick, S., et al. 2009. Postmenopausal hormone therapy and regional brain volumes: The WHIMS–MRI Study. *Neurology, 72* (2), 135–142.

Simon, J., et al. 2001. Effect of estrogen plus progestin on risk for biliary tract surgery in postmenopausal women with coronary artery disease. The Heart and Estrogen/progestin Replacement Study (HERS). *Ann. Int. Med., 135* (7), 493-501.

Sites, C., et al. 2005. The effect of hormone replacement therapy on body composition, body fat distribution, and insulin sensitivity in menopausal women: A randomized, double-blind, placebo-controlled trial. *J. Clin. Endocrinol. Metab., 95* (5), 2701–2707.

Ursin, G., et al. 2004. Post-treatment change in serum estrone predicts mammographic percent density changes in women who received combination estrogen and progestin in the Postmenopausal Estrogen/Progestin Interventions (PEPI) trial. *J. Clin. Oncol., 22* (14), 2842–2848.

Effects of estrogen or estrogen/progestin regimens on heart disease risk factors in postmenopausal women. The Postmenopausal Estrogen/Progestin Interventions (PEPI) Trial. The Writing Group for the PEPI Trial. *JAMA* 1995 Jan 18;273(3):199-208.

Black Cohosh

Einbond LS, Shimizu M, Xiao D, et al. Growth inhibitory activity of extracts and purified components of black cohosh on human breast cancer cells. *Breast Cancer Res Treat.* 2004; 83(3):221–231.

Affects of Soy on Breasts

Allred CD, Ju YH, Allred KF, Chang J, Helferich WG. Dietary genistin stimulates growth of estrogen-dependent breast cancer tumors similar to that observed with genistein. *Carcinogenesis* 2001 Oct; 22(10):1667-73.

Dees C, Foster JS, Ahamed S, Wimalasena J. Dietary estrogens stimulate human breast cells to enter the cell cycle. *Environmental Health Perspective.* 1997 Apr 105 Suppl 3 633-6.

de Lemos ML. Effects of soy phytoestrogens genistein and daidzein on breast cancer growth. *Ann Pharmacother* 2001 Sep; 35(9):1118-21.

Di Virgilio AL, Iwami K, Watjen W, Kahl R, Degen GH.Genotoxicity of the isoflavones genistein, daidzein and equol in V79 cells. *Toxicol Lett.* 2004 Jun 15; 151(1):151-62.

Hsieh CY, Santell RC, Haslam SZ, Helferich WG. Estrogenic effects of genistein on the growth of estrogen receptor-positive human breast cancer (MCF-7) cells in vitro and in vivo. *Cancer Research.* 1998 Sep 1 58:17 3833-8.

Ju YH, Allred CD, Allred KF, Karko KL, Doerge DR, Helferich WG. Physiological concentrations of dietary genistein dose-dependently stimulate growth of estrogen-dependent human breast cancer (MCF-7) tumors implanted in athymic nude mice. *J Nutr.* 2001 Nov; 131(11):2957-62.

Metzler M, Kulling SE, Pfeiffer E and Jacobs E. Z Genotoxicity Of Estrogens. *Lebensm Unters Forsch A.* 1998, 206: 367-73.

Petrakis NL et al. Stimulatory influence of soy protein isolate on breast secretion in pre- and postmenopausal women. *Cancer Epid Bio Prev.* 1996; 5: 785-794.

Trock BJ, Hilakivi-Clarke L, Clarke R. Meta-analysis of soy intake and breast cancer risk. *J Natl Cancer Inst.* 2006 Apr 5; 98(7):430-1.

Soy intake may be associated with a small reduction in breast cancer risk. However, this result should be interpreted with caution due to potential exposure misclassification, confounding, and lack of a dose response. Given these caveats and results of some experimental studies that suggest adverse effects from soy constituents, recommendations for high-dose isoflavone supplementation to prevent breast cancer or prevent its recurrence are premature.

Flaxseeds

McCann SE, Muti P, Vito D, Edge S. Dietary lignan intakes and risk of pre- and postmenopausal breast cancer. *BInt J Cancer.* 2004 Sep 1; 111(3):440-3.

Boccardo F et al: Serum enterolactone levels and the risk of breast cancer in women with palpable cysts, Eur *J Cancer.* 2004 Jan; 40(1):84-9.

SS. Pruthi, S.L. Thompson, P.J. Novotny, D.L. Barton, L.A. Kottschade, A.D. Tan, J.A. Sloan, C.L. Loprinzi. *Pilot* Evaluation of Flaxseed for the Management of Hot Flashes. *Journal of the Society for Integrative Oncology.* Volume 5, Number 3, doi: 10.2310/7200.2007.007

CHAPTER 3

Xenoestrogens

Tapiero H, Ba GN et al. Estrogens and environmental estrogens. *Biomed Pharmacother*. 2002 Feb; 56(1):36–44.

Yanick, P. *Prohormone Nutrition*, Montclair, NJ: Longevity Institute International, 1998; p. 358.

Failure of Synthetic Hormones to Initiate Normal Response

Yanick, P. *Prohormone Nutrition*, Montclair, NJ: Longevity Institute International, 1998; p. 358.

Causes of Progesterone Deficiency

Lee, John R., *What Your Doctor May Not Tell You About Menopause*. Warner Books, May, 1996.

Smith, P. *HRT: The Answers*, Traverse City, MI: Healthy Living Books, Inc, 2003; p. 29.

Progesterone
Ovulation

Marshall JC, Eagleson CA, McCartney CR. Hypothalamic dysfunction. *Mol Cell Endocrinol* 2001 Oct 25;183(1-2):29-32.

Administration of progesterone can slow GnRH pulse secretion, favor FSH secretion and induce follicular maturation. Thus, the ability to change the pattern of GnRH secretion is an important factor in the maintenance of cyclic ovulation, and loss of this function leads to anovulation and amenorrhea.

Progesterone
Nausea and Vomiting in Pregnancy, PMS, Dysmenorrhea

Mabray CR, Burditt ML, Martin TL, Jaynes CR, Hayes JR. Treatment of common gynecologic-endocrinologic symptoms by allergy management procedures. *Obstet Gynecol* 1982 May; 59(5):560-4.

The technique of managing allergies by optimum-dose (provocative neutralization) testing and treatment using aqueous progesterone has been studied in 132 women having progesterone-related symptoms due to the menstrual cycle, pregnancy, or exogenous hormone administration. When extremely small doses of progesterone (0.0016 mg or below, up to maximum of 2.5 mg) were administered following determination of specific dose requirement by skin testing, startlingly rapid and effective clearing of symptoms was observed. With these individualized doses, symptoms cleared completely or almost completely within 30 minutes in the majority of patients. A single-blind technique was employed to rule out placebo effect. Some common problems found to respond well to the procedure were nausea and vomiting during pregnancy (100%), premenstrual syndrome (96%), and dysmenorrhea (84%).

Progesterone
Fetal Brain Development

Dalton K. The effect of Progesterone and progestogens on the fetus. *Neuropharmacology* 1981; 20(12B):1267-9.

This article looks at the differing effects of Progesterone and synthetic progestogens on the fetus. Of note in this article is evidence that progesterone supplementation may reduce episodes of pre-eclampsia. Synthetic progestogen supplementation during pregnancy may produce a variety of side effects. Several references are made to articles documenting cases of masculinization of external genitalia in female babies. There are two known cases of true hermaphroditism and several cases of behavioral problems developing in adolescent girls whose mothers took oral synthetic progestogens during pregnancy. More problematic may be administration of oral estrogen-progestogen preparations. Side effects may include spina bifida, esophageal anomalies, heart defects and limb reduction deformities.

Dalton K. Prenatal progesterone and educational attainments. *Br J Psychiatry 1976; 129:438-42.*

This study compares educational attainments of 34 children whose mothers received prenatal progesterone with 37 normal and 12 toxemic controls. Results at ages 17-24 showed that progesterone children were more likely to continue schooling after 16 years, a higher number left school with 'O' and 'A' level grades and more obtained entrance to university. The best academic results were found for children whose mothers had received over 5 grams of progesterone for a minimum of eight weeks, with treatment beginning before week sixteen.

Dalton, K., *The British Journal of Psychiatry* (1968) 114: 1377-1382.

J.M. Reinish, *The Female Patient*, April, 1978, p.87.

Lee, John R., Zava, David, *What Your Doctor May Not Tell You About Breast Cancer*, Warner Books, 2002; p.94.

Natural progesterone increases a child's IQ, typically by around 35 points and produces personalities that are more "independent, individualistic, self-assured, self-sufficient and sensitive".

Progesterone
Effect on Estrogen

Nahoul K, Dehennin L, Jondet M, Roger M.Profiles of plasma estrogens, progesterone and their metabolites after oral or vaginal administration of estradiol or progesterone. *Maturitas.* 1993; 16:185–202.

Progesterone is permissive for the action of estradiol, increases circulating levels of estradiol possibly allowing for reduced dosing of estradiol.

Progesterone
PMS

Dennerstein L, Spencer-Gardner C, Gotts G, Brown JB, Smith MA, Burrows GD. Progesterone and the premenstrual syndrome: a double blind crossover trial. *Br Med J.* (Clin Res Ed) 1985; 290(6482): 1617-21.

*In this double-blind, placebo-controlled, randomized, crossover trial, oral micronized progesterone demonstrated effectiveness in alleviating premenstrual complaints. Twenty-three women completed a Beck, et al depression inventory, Moos's menstrual distress questionnaire, Spielberger, et al state anxiety inventory, and daily symptom diary before and during each treatment. There was an overall benefit of treatment for all variables, except positive moods, restlessness, and interest in sex. For most parameters, maximum benefit was seen within the first month of treatment, demonstrating an effectiveness of progesterone as a viable treatment option for women with PMS. ***

Magill PJ.Hoechst UK Ltd., Hounslow, Middlesex. Investigation of the efficacy of progesterone pessaries in the relief of symptoms of premenstrual syndrome. progesterone Study Group. *Br J Gen Pract.* 1995 Nov; 45(400):589-93.

*In this study, progesterone, given as pessaries by vaginal or rectal administration, was more effective than placebo in the relief of symptoms of premenstrual syndrome in a population of patients selected by strict entry criteria.***

Wyatt K, Dimmock P, Jones P, Obhrai M, O'Brien S. Efficacy of progesterone and progestogens in management of premenstrual syndrome: systematic review. *BMJ.* 2001; 323(7316):776-80.

*This systematic review of published studies of progesterone or progestogens for treatment of PMS found a small positive effect of oral micronized progesterone over placebo in the 3 trials that studied this. No published studies of progesterone cream were found. A statistically, but not clinically, significant improvement was seen with progestogen treatment.**

Yonkers K. Review: progesterone or progestogens lead to a marginal reduction in premenstrual syndrome symptoms. *Evid Based Ment Health.* 2002; 5(2):56.

*The author conducted an analysis of randomized, double blind, placebo-controlled studies of progesterone or progestins in women diagnosed with PMS. Oral micronized progesterone and the progestogens MPA, norethisterone and dydrogesterone, all showed a marginal benefit over placebo in symptom reduction.**

Estrogen Dominance in PMS

Barnhardt, K. T., et al. 1995. A clinician's guide to the premenstrual syndrome. *Medical Clinician of North America.* 79:1457-1472.

Facchinetti, F. et al. 1983. Estradiol/progesterone imbalance and the premenstural syndrome. *Lancet* 2:13-2.

Munday, MR, Brush, MG, Taylor, RW. Correlations between progesterone, oestradiol and aldosterone levels in the premenstrual syndrome. *Clin Endocrino.l* (Oxf) 1981 Jan; 14(1):1-9.

All the PMS patients were ovulatory but the progesterone values from days −9 to −5 premenstrually were significantly lower than the control values. The oestradiol levels in the PMS patients were higher than in control subjects over the last 4 days of the cycle suggesting estrogen dominance correlates with PMS.

Progesterone
Endometriosis

Maginnis G, Wilk, J. Assessment of progestin-only therapy for endometriosis in macaque. *J Med Primatol.* 2008 Feb; 37 Suppl 1:52-5.

Progesterone
Hot Flashes, Night Sweats and Menopausal Symptoms

Leonetti HB, Longo S, Anasti, JN. Transdermal Progesterone cream for vasomotor symptoms and postmenopausal bone loss. *Obstet Gynecol.* 1999; 94(2):225-8.

In this randomized controlled trial, 102 menopausal women were treated with topical Progesterone (Pro-gest®, 20 mg daily) or placebo and monitored for 1 year. Improvement in vasomotor symptoms was seen in 83% of the women in the treatment group who had experienced hot flashes, compared to 19% in the placebo group (p< .001). There was no difference noted in bone mineral densities between groups after one year. All women studied received a daily multivitamin and 1200 mg calcium.*

Stephenson, K. et. al. Transdermal progesterone significantly relieves menopausal symptoms in postmenopausal women assessed by Greene Climacteric Scale scores. *Blood.* (Annual Meeting Abstracts) 2004 104. Abstract 5318.

Progesterone
As a Diuretic (Potassium Sparing)

Miller WL., Chrousos GP., The Adrenal Cortex. *Endocrinology and Metabolism.* 4th ed. McGraw-Hill, Inc. 2001: 435.

M Quinkler, B Myer, C Bumke-Vogt, *European Journal of Endocrinology.* 2002; 146:789-800.

Progesterone
Breast Health

Campagnoli C, Abba C, Ambroggio S, Peris C. Pregnancy, Progesterone and progestins in relation to breast cancer risk. *J Steroid Biochem Mol Biol.* 2005; 97(5):441-50.

The authors review recent findings that show that the production of Progesterone during pregnancy and the use of bioidentical progesterone in hormone therapy do not increase breast cancer risk, and can even protect against the development of breast cancer.*

Chang KJ, Lee TT, Linares-Cruz G, Fournier S, de Lignieres B. Influences of percutaneous administration of estradiol and progesterone on human breast epithelial cell cycle in vivo. *Fertil Steril.* 1995; 63(4):785-91.

The effect of transdermal estradiol (1.5 mg), transdermal progesterone (25 mg), and combined transdermal estradiol and progesterone (1.5 mg and 25 mg) on human breast epithelial cell cycles was evaluated in vivo. Results demonstrated that estradiol significantly increases cell proliferation, while progesterone significantly decreases cell replication below that observed with placebo. Transdermal progesterone was also shown to reduce estradiol-induced proliferation.*

Cowan LD, Gordis L, Tonascia JA, Jones GS. Breast cancer incidence in women with a history of progesterone deficiency. *Am J Epidemiol.*1981; 114:209-17.

1083 infertile women were followed for 14-34 years. Those who were deficient in progesterone showed a five-fold greater incidence of premenopausal breast cancer.*

Desreux J, Kebers F, Noel A, Francart D, Van Cauwenberge H, Heinen V, Thomas JL, Bernard AM, Paris J, Delansorne R, Foidart

JM. Progesterone receptor activation - an alternative to SERMs in breast cancer. *Eur J Cancer* 2000; 36 Suppl 4:S90-1.

This review emphasizes Progesterone's role in supporting healthy breast homeostasis and opposing the proliferative effects of estradiol in the breast, unlike synthetic progestins.

Foidart JM, Colin C, Denoo X, Desreux J, Beliard A, Fournier S, de Lignieres B. Estradiol and Progesterone regulate the proliferation of human breast epithelial cells. *Fertil Steril.* 1998; 69(5):963-9.

In this double-blind randomized study, to evaluate the effects of estrogen and progesterone on normal breast cells, 40 postmenopausal women received daily topical application of a gel containing either placebo, estradiol, progesterone, or estradiol + progesterone for two weeks prior to esthetic breast surgery or the excision of a benign breast lesion. The results showed that increased estrogen concentration increased the number of cycling epithelial cells, whereas exposure to progesterone for 14 days reduced the estrogen-induced proliferation of normal breast epithelial cells.

Formby B, Wiley TS. Progesterone inhibits growth and induces apoptosis in breast cancer cells: inverse effects on Bcl-2 and p53. *Ann Clin Lab Sci.* 1998; 28(6):360-9.

This study explored the mechanism by which Progesterone inhibits breast cancer cell proliferation (growth). In progesterone receptor positive T47-D breast cancer cells, the mechanism of apoptosis appeared to be through the regulation of the genes p53 and bcl-2 by progesterone. These genes control the apoptotic process. It was demonstrated that at progesterone levels that approximate the third trimester of pregnancy, there was a strong antiproliferative effect in at least 2 breast cancer cell lines.*

Formby B, Wiley TS. Bcl-2, survivin and variant CD44 v7-v10 are downregulated and p53 is upregulated in breast cancer cells by

Progesterone: inhibition of cell growth and induction of apoptosis. *Mol Cell Biochem.* 1999; 202(1-2):53-61.

This study sought to elucidate the mechanism by which progesterone inhibits the proliferation of breast cancer cells. Utilizing breast cancer cell lines with and without progesterone receptors (T47-D and MDA-231, respectively) in vitro, the authors looked at apoptosis (programmed cell death) in response to progesterone exposure as a possible mechanism. The genetic markers for apoptosis - p53, bcl-2 and surviving, were utilized to determine whether or not the cells underwent apoptosis. The results demonstrated that progesterone does produce a strong antiproliferative effect on breast cancer cell lines containing progesterone receptors, and induced apoptosis. The relatively high levels of progesterone utilized were similar to those seen during the third trimester of human pregnancy.*

Fournier A, Berrino F, Clavel-Chapelon F. Unequal risks for breast cancer associated with different hormone replacement therapies: results from the E3N cohort study. *Breast Cancer Res Treat.* 2008; 107(1):103-11.

This large multicenter study in France followed 80,377 postmenopausal women for up to 12 years, and looked in particular at whether the type of progestogen used in combination with estrogen made a difference to the risk of developing breast cancer in those women who used hormone replacement therapy (HRT). The estrogen in HRT is primarily transdermal estradiol in France. Compared with those women who did not use HRT at all, women using estrogen alone had a 1.29-fold increased risk of developing breast cancer; women using estrogen plus natural Progesterone had the same risk as women using no HRT. In women using synthetic progestins in combination with estrogen, the particular progestin used made a difference to breast cancer risk; women using dydrogesterone had a 1.16-fold increased risk of breast cancer, but those using other progestins had a 1.69-fold increased risk of breast cancer, compared to women not using HRT. The authors note that dydrogesterone is *the progestin most similar to natural progesterone in its chemical structure and pharmacological effects. ***

Fournier A, Berrino F, Riboli E, Avenel V, Clavel-Chapelon F. Breast cancer risk in relation to different types of hormone replacement therapy in the E3N-EPIC cohort. *Int J Cancer.* 2005; 114(3):448-54.

*Combined HRT with estrogen (either oral or transdermal) and synthetic progestins was found to carry a significantly increased risk of breast cancer compared with estrogens plus oral micronized Progesterone. In fact, no increase in breast cancer risk was seen in the estrogen plus oral micronized progesterone group compared with estrogen alone. This large multicenter study therefore suggests that there is a dramatic difference between the effects of bioidentical progesterone versus synthetic progestins on breast cancer risk.***

Greendale GA, Reboussin BA, Slone S, Wasilauskas C, Pike MC, Ursin G. Postmenopausal hormone therapy and change in mammographic density. *J Natl Cancer Inst.* 2003; 95(1):30-7.

*Greater mammographic density was associated with the use of estrogen/progestin combination therapy, although the micronized progesterone containing arm appeared to induce a smaller increase than that with MPA.***

Holtorf K. The Bioidentical Hormone Debate: Are Bioidentical Hormones (Estradiol, Estriol, and Progesterone) Safer or More Efficacious than Commonly Used Synthetic Versions in Hormone Replacement Therapy? *Postgrad Med.* 2009; 121(1):1-13.

This literature review presents the substantial evidence for the safety and efficacy of bioidentical hormone therapy, including estradiol, estriol, and Progesterone, which shows that it presents lower risks for breast cancer and cardiovascular disease than synthetic or animal-derived hormones. Studies show that progestins have a number of negative effects on the cardiovascular system and an *association with breast cancer risk that can be avoided by using bioidentical progesterone.**

Kaaks R, Berrino F, Key T, Rinaldi S, Dossus L, Biessy C, Secreto G, Amiano P, Bingham S, Boeing H, Bueno de Mesquita HB, Chang-Claude J, Clavel-Chapelon F, Fournier A, et al. Serum sex steroids in premenopausal women and breast cancer risk within the European Prospective Investigation into Cancer and Nutrition (EPIC). *J Natl Cancer Inst.* 2005; 97:755-65.

In this large multicenter study, higher serum Progesterone levels were associated with a significant reduction in breast cancer risk.*

Laidlaw IJ, Clarke RB, Howell A, Owen AW, Potten CS, Anderson E. The proliferation of normal breast tissue implanted into athymic nude mice is stimulated by estrogen, but not by progesterone. *Endocrinology.* 1995; 136(1):164-71.

Normal human breast tissue was implanted subcutaneously into athymic nude mice. The mice were then treated with estradiol or progesterone such that serum levels approximated those seen in normal menstruating women. Immunocytochemical measures were made of proliferative activity and steroid receptor expression of the tissue implants. It was found that physiologic levels of estradiol significantly stimulated the proliferation of human breast epithelial cells and increased progesterone receptor expression 10-20-fold. Progesterone failed to affect proliferation alone or after estradiol priming.*

Lin VC, Ng EH, Aw SE, Tan MG, Ng EH, Chan VS, Ho GH. Progestins inhibit the growth of MDA-MB-231 cells transfected with Progesterone receptor complementary DNA. *Clin Cancer Res.* 1999; 5(2):395-403.

Progesterone is mainly thought to exert its effects via the estrogen-dependent progesterone receptor (PR), the effects of which may be overshadowed by the presence of estrogen. In order to study *the independent effects of progesterone on breast cancer cell lines, PR expression vectors were transfected into a PR and ER negative cell line (MDA-MB-231). The growth of these cells was then studied in response to progesterone and several progestins. Progesterone was found to significantly inhibit DNA synthesis and cell growth in a dose-dependant fashion. The results of this study indicate that progesterone and progestins independent of estrogen have an antiproliferative effect on breast cancer cells via the progesterone receptor. This suggests a possible role in the treatment of PR negative breast cancer via re-activation of the PR receptor.**

Lee, John R., Zava, David, *What Your Doctor May Not Tell You About Breast Cancer*, Warner Books, 2002; p.94.

Malet C, Spritzer P, Guillaumin D, Kuttenn F. Progesterone effect on cell growth, ultrastructural aspect and estradiol receptors of normal human breast epithelial (HBE) cells in culture. *J Steroid Biochem Mol Bio.l* 2000; 73: 171-81.

In a culture system, progesterone was found to have an inhibitory effect on breast cell growth. When given following estradiol (E2), it limited the stimulatory effect of E2 on cell growth.*

Mauvais-Jarvis P, Kuttenn F, Gompel A. Antiestrogen action of progesterone in breast tissue. *Horm Res* 1987;28(2-4):212-8.

In a review of international literature on the cellular effects of progesterone on both normal breast cells and breast cancer cell lines, the authors conclude that most data indicate progesterone and progestins have an antiestrogenic effect on the breast, as reflected in the decrease in estradiol receptor content, the decrease in cell proliferation, and an increase in a marker of cell differentiation, 17 beta-hydroxysteroid activity, which is mediated by the progesterone receptor.*

Missmer SA, Eliassen AH, Barbieri RL, Hankinson SE. Endogenous estrogen, androgen, and progesterone concentrations and breast cancer risk among postmenopausal women. *J Natl Cancer Inst.* 2004; 96(24):1856-65.

Blood progesterone levels were found not to be related to breast cancer risk in this first study to investigate this in postmenopausal women. The occurrence of progesterone receptor positive tumors was the tumor type most strongly affected by all the circulating steroid hormones measured except for progesterone. Higher levels of endogenous estrogens and androgens were significantly correlated with increasing breast cancer incidence. This suggests that circulating natural progesterone does not increase breast cancer risk.*

Mohr PE, Wang DY, Gregory WM, Richards MA, Fentiman IS. Serum Progesterone and prognosis in operable breast cancer. *Br J Cancer.* 1996;73:1552-5.

Higher blood levels of Progesterone measured during surgical treatment of breast cancers were associated with significantly better survival, especially in women who were node-positive (P<0.01). There was no significant relationship between estradiol levels and survival. This study demonstrated that a higher level of progesterone at time of excision is associated with improved prognosis in women with operable breast cancer.

Plu-Bureau G, Le MG, Thalabard JC, Sitruk-Ware R, Mauvais-Jarvis P. Percutaneous progesterone use and risk of breast cancer: results from a French cohort study of premenopausal women with benign breast disease. *Cancer Detect Prev.*1999; 23(4):290-6.

This cohort study followed 1150 premenopausal French women diagnosed with benign breast disease. Topical progesterone cream, a common treatment for mastalgia in Europe, had been prescribed to 58% of the women. Follow-up accumulated 12,462 person-years. There was no association noted between progesterone cream use and breast cancer risk. Furthermore, women who had used both progesterone cream and an oral progestogen had a significant decrease in breast cancer risk (RR= 0.5) as compared to women who did *not use progesterone cream. There was no significant difference in the risk of breast cancer in percutaneous progesterone users versus nonusers among oral progestogen users. These results suggest there are no deleterious effects caused by percutaneous progesterone use in women with benign breast disease.* *

Santos SJ, Aupperlee MD, Xie J, Durairaj S, Miksicek R, Conrad SE, Leipprandt JR, Tan YS, Schwartz RC, Haslam SZ. Progesterone receptor A-regulated gene expression in mammary organoid cultures. *J Steroid Biochem Mol Biol.* 2009; 115(3-5):161-72.

This experimental study used breast cells from mice, cultured in vitro. First, the behavior of the cells was compared after exposure to either Progesterone or the synthetic progestin, promogestone. After seeing similar proliferation with both progestogens, they then went on to conduct gene expression studies (again in the mouse mammary cells) using only the promogestone. They found that certain genes were activated by the promogestone, and these were regulated by progesterone receptor A, which is increased relative to progesterone receptor B in more aggressive breast cancers in humans. The researchers imply that the expression of these genes in the cultured mouse breast cells may translate to growth-promoting actions of progesterone in the breast tissue in humans. However, human tissue was not studied here, and the mouse cells under investigation were in an environment very different to that under which they would be growing in the intact mouse. Any conclusions regarding the possibility that progesterone in itself could promote breast cancer in a living human can, therefore, not be inferred from this study. In addition, synthetic progestins are already known to have very different actions to those of progesterone itself in clinical studies. Progesterone has not been shown to cause or exacerbate breast cancer in women; on the contrary, it has been found in clinical studies to be associated with a lower breast cancer risk. *

Progesterone
Breast Pain and Fibrocystic Breast Disease

Nappi C, Affinito P, Di Carlo C, Esposito G, Montemagno U. Double-blind controlled trial of Progesterone vaginal cream treatment for cyclical mastodynia in women with benign breast disease. *J Endocrinol Invest*. 1992; 15(11):801-6.

Eighty regularly menstruating women with mastodynia were studied to evaluate the clinical effectiveness of vaginally administered micronized Progesterone. Subjects were randomly assigned to one of two groups, with all participating in a control cycle prior to treatment. One group received 4 grams of vaginal cream containing 2.5% natural progesterone for six cycles from day 19 to day 25 of the cycle. The other group was similarly treated with placebo. Both subjective reporting on a daily basis and clinical examination revealed a significant reduction in breast pain, defined as 50% reduction, in 64.9% of subjects receiving progesterone and 22.2% of subjects receiving placebo. Effects of breast nodularity were not significant. No side effects were detected.

Plu-Bureau G, Le M, Thalabard J, et. al. Topical progesterone in 1150 women with fibrocystic breasts indicated no increased risk of cancer. *Cancer Detect Prev*. 1999; 23:290-296.

Progesterone
Ovarian Cancer

Yu S, Lee M, Shin S, Park J. Apoptosis induced by progesterone in human ovarian cancer cell line SNU-840. *J Cell Biochem*. 2001;82(3):445-51.

Researchers demonstrated that progesterone caused inhibition of growth of epithelial ovarian cancer cells and elicited apotosis.

Progesterone
Endometrial Cancer

Donghai Dai, Douglas M. Wolf, Elizabeth S. Litman, Michael J. White, and Kimberly K. Leslie. Progesterone Inhibits Human Endometrial Cancer Cell Growth and Invasiveness: Down-Regulation of Cellular Adhesion Molecules through Progesterone B Receptors. *Cancer Res.* 2002 62: 881-886.

Progesterone
Osteoporosis

Barengolts EL, Gajardo HF, Rosol TJ, D'Anza JJ, Pena M, Botsis J, Kukreja SC. Effects of progesterone on postovariectomy bone loss in aged rats. *J Bone Miner Res.* 1990 Nov;5(11):1143-7.

Bowman BM, Miller SC. Elevated progesterone during pseudo-pregnancy may prevent bone loss associated with low estrogen. *J Bone Miner Res.* 1996 Jan; 11(1):15-21.

Burnett CC, Reddi AH. Influence of estrogen and progesterone on matrix-induced endochondral bone formation. *Calcif Tissue Int.* 1983 Jul; 35(4-5): 609-14.

Gronowicz GA, McCarthy M-B. Glucocorticoids inhibit the attachment of osteoblasts to bone extracellular matrix proteins and decrease B1-integrin levels. *Endocrinology.* 1995; 136:598-608.

Progesterone binding to glucocorticoid receptors also may modulate bone loss. Glucocorticoids cause bone loss by blocking osteocalcin synthesis and preventing the attachment of osteoblasts to matrix proteins. Studies indicate that progesterone exerts an anti-glucocorticoid effect.*

Lee JR; Is Natural Progesterone the Missing Link in Osteoporosis Prevention and Treatment? *Medical Hypothesis.* 1991; 35:316-318.

Lee JR. Osteoporosis reversal; the role of progesterone. *International Clinical Nutrition Review* 1990; 10(3):384-91.

Luo XH, Liao EY. Progesterone differentially regulates the membrane-type matrix metalloproteinase-1 (MT1 -MMP) compartment of proMMP-2 activation in MG-63 cells. *Horm Metab Res.* 2001 Jul; 33(7):383-8.

Osteoblast-derived matrix metalloproteinases (MMPs) are considered to play a crucial role in bone formation and initiation of bone resorption by degrading the bone matrix. Progesterone may contribute to its actions on bone formation.*

MacNamara P, Loughrey HC. Progesterone receptor A and B isoform expression in human osteoblasts. *Calcif Tissue Int.* 1998; 63:39-46.

Bone-forming cells are physiologically influenced by progesterone.

Prior, JC, Vigna Y, Alojado N. *Canadian Journal of Obstetrics/ Gynecology and Women's Health Care.* 1991; 3(4):178-84.

In this review article, the authors propose that cyclic progesterone both prevents bone loss and acts as a bone-builder. The studies discussed focus on abnormal menstrual cycles as an important risk factor for osteoporotic fractures. Their conclusion is that the first step in preventing osteoporosis is treating ovulation disorders.*

Prior, JC. Progesterone as a Bone-trophic hormone. *Endocr Rev* 1990; 11(2):386-98.

Transdermal progesterone supplementation with and without conjugated estrogens was evaluated in a clinical setting using 100 women aged 38 to 83 years. The average time from onset of menopause was 16 years. 63 women were followed for three years with dual photon absorptiometry. Treatment also included dietary changes, nutritional supplements, and exercise. All individuals followed showed an increase in bone mineral density over the three *years, with the greatest increase occurring in the first year. There was no difference noted between estrogen/progesterone and progesterone only groups. Subjective changes included increased libido, diminished hot flushes, reduced joint pain, and increased mobility and energy. No side effects were noted during treatment protocol.**

Prior JC, Vigna YM, Schecter MI, Burgess AE. Spinal Bone loss and ovulatory disturbances. *N Engl J Med* 1990; 323(18):1221-7.

A review of the available data indicates that progesterone acts to promote bone metabolism. It appears to be independent of estrogen by either acting directly at progesterone receptors, or indirectly through competition at glucocorticoid receptors in the osteoblasts.*

Progesterone
Wrinkles

Holzer, G.; Riegler, E.; Hönigsmann, H.; Farokhnia, S.; Schmidt, B. Effects and side-effects of 2% progesterone cream on the skin of peri- and postmenopausal women: results from a double-blind, vehicle-controlled, randomized study. *British Journal of Dermatology.* 2005; 153 (3): 626-634(9).

This 16-week study in 40 women, conducted by Dr. Holzer and colleagues, evaluated the effects of 2% progesterone cream on function and texture of the skin in women at or after menopause. The study design was robust: double-blind, placebo-controlled, and randomized. The results showed 23% increase in skin firmness, 29% reduction in wrinkle count near the eye and almost 10% reduction of the depth of laugh lines. No serious side-effects were observed.*

Progesterone
Asthma

Beynon HL, Garbett ND, Barnes PJ. Severe premenstrual exacerbations of asthma: effect of intramuscular progesterone. *Lancet.* 1988 Aug 13; 2(8607):370-2.

Three patients with severe premenstrual exacerbations of asthma are reported. None had responded to conventional treatment, including high-dose corticosteroids. In all cases there was a striking fall premenstrually in peak flow rate. The addition of intramuscular progesterone (100 mg daily in two cases and 600 mg twice a week in one) to the regimen eliminated the premenstrual dips in peak flow, and daily doses of prednisolone were reduced in the three patients.

Progesterone
Heart Health

Bagis T, Gokcel A, Zeyneloglu HB, Tarim E, Kilicdag EB, Haydardedeoglu B. The effects of short-term medroxyprogesterone acetate and micronized progesterone on glucose metabolism and lipid profiles in patients with polycystic ovary syndrome: a prospective randomized study. *J Clin Endocrinol Metab* 2002; 87(10):4536-40.

This randomized prospective study evaluated and compared the effects of ten days treatment with oral and vaginal micronized progesterone (MP) and medroxyprogesterone acetate (MPA) on glucose metabolism, lipid profiles, and hormonal parameters in 28 patients with polycystic ovary syndrome (PCOS). Oral MPA and oral MP decreased luteinizing hormone and total testosterone levels. There was no change in hormonal parameters with vaginal MP. Basal insulin decreased and insulin sensitivity increased significantly in the oral MPA group. Low density lipoprotein cholesterol (LDL) and lipoprotein (a) levels decreased only in the MPA group. This study concluded that MPA and oral MP may increase insulin sensitivity in patients with PCOS. Vaginal MP had no effect on glucose metabolism and lipid profiles.

Chataigneau T, Zerr M, Chataigneau M, Hudlett F, Hirn C, Pernot F, Schini-Kerth VB. Chronic treatment with progesterone but not medroxyprogesterone acetate restores the endothelial control of vascular tone in the mesenteric artery of ovariectomized rats. *Menopause.* 2004; 11(3):255-63.

This study helps explain the more beneficial effects on the cardiovascular system of progesterone compared with MPA because of its enhancement of the protective effects of endothelial cells on the arterial walls.*

Chang HY, et al. Different role of endothelium/nitric oxide in 17 B-estradiol and progesterone-induced relaxation in rat arteries. *Life Sci.* 2001; 69:1609-1617.

Progesterone dilates coronary arteries by increasing nitric oxide.

Crews JK, Khalil RA. Antagonistic effects of 17B-estradiol, progesterone, and testosterone on Ca++ entry mechanisms of coronary vasoconstriction. *Arterioscler Thromb Vasc Biol.* 1999; 19:1034-1040.

Researchers have found that progesterone reduces platelet aggregation via the enhancement of nitric oxide, which is an endothelium-derived relaxing factor. One study showed progesterone actually caused coronary relaxation by inhibiting Ca++ mobilization into coronary smooth muscle.

Gillson GR, Zava DT. A perspective on HRT for women: picking up the pieces after the Women's Health Initiative trial - Part 2. *Int J Pharm Compounding.* 2003; 7(5):330-8.

The authors review clinical evidence for the benefits of bioidentical progesterone over synthetic progestins. While both protect the uterine lining from proliferation caused by estrogens, progesterone has beneficial effects on Cardiovascular health. The synergy between progesterone and estradiol, each "turning on" the other's receptors, has the added benefit of allowing the estradiol dosage to be reduced. Oral and transdermal dosing of bioidentical progesterone are discussed.*

Hermsmeyer RK, Thompson TL, Pohost GM, Kaski JC. Cardiovascular effects of medroxyprogesterone acetate and progesterone:

a case of mistaken identity? *Nat Clin Pract Cardiovasc Med.* 2008; 5(7):387-95.

The authors present the current state of knowledge about the cardiovascular effects of progesterone compared to medroxyprogesterone acetate (MPA). They caution that the beneficial effects of natural progesterone on cardiovascular risk have been obscured by the negative results of large trials involving hormone therapy that included MPA, in which cardiac risk was seen to increase. The review covers the evidence that natural progesterone actually improves cardiovascular function, and compares oral and transdermal delivery.*

Hermsmeyer RK, Mishra RG, Pavcnik D, Uchida B, Axthelm MK, Stanczyk FZ, Burry KA, Illingworth DR, Kaski JC, Nordt FJ. Prevention of coronary hyperreactivity in pre-atherogenic menopausal rhesus monkeys by transdermal progesterone. *Arterioscler Thromb Vasc Biol.* 2004;24(5):955-61.

Previous studies by Hermsmeyer, et al demonstrated a reduction of coronary reactivity in response to sub-physiological levels of progesterone in non-atherogenic monkeys. In this study, the authors sought to determine if transdermal progesterone cream conferred coronary vascular protection in surgically menopausal pre-atherosclerotic rhesus monkeys. Compared with monkeys receiving placebo cream (n= 5), treated monkeys (n= 7) experienced reduced Lipoprotein (a) levels, and an attenuation of coronary vasoconstriction, which was artificially stimulated by intracoronary serotonin plus U46619. Coronary hyperreactivity is a component of coronary artery disease and was demonstrated in this study to be prevented in pre-atherosclerotic primates by progesterone cream treatment.

Jiang C, Sarrel PM, Lindsay DC, et al. Progesterone induces endothelium-independent relaxation of rabbit coronary artery in vivo. *Eur J Pharmacol.* 1992; 211:163-167.

Lee WS, Harder JA. Progesterone inhibits arterial smooth muscle cell proliferation. *Nat Med.* 1997; 3:1005-1008.

Progesterone inhibits atheroscleroticplaque formation.

Marianne Canonico, PhD, et al. Hormone Therapy and Venous Thromboembolism Among Postmenopausal Women, Impact of the Route of Estrogen Administration and Progestogens: The ESTHER Study. *Circulation.* 2007 Feb 20; 115(7):840-5.

Bioidentical progesterone when used with estrogen decreases risk of blood clots 30 percent.

Mather KJ, Norman EG, Prior JC, Elliott TG. Preserved forearm endothelial responses with acute exposure to Progesterone: A randomized cross-over trial of 17-beta estradiol, progesterone, and 17-beta estradiol with progesterone in healthy menopausal women. *J Clin Endocrinol Metab* 2000; 85(12):4644-9.

Regularly menstruating women enjoy relative protection from cardiovascular disease. Until recently, this has been attributed to the function of estrogen, despite the fact that Progesterone is also present. This study evaluated the differing acute effects of 17-beta estradiol alone, 17-beta estradiol with progesterone and just progesterone alone on endothelial function in a randomized crossover trial. Endothelial function was evaluated via endothelium dependent and independent forearm blood flow (FBF) using venous occlusion plethysmography. Flow responses were measured during brachial artery infusions achieving physiological levels of E2, E2 + P4, or P4 respectively along with either acetylcholine (an endothelium-dependent vasodilator), or sodium nitroprusside (an endothelium-independent vasodilator) in 27 healthy menopausal women with no cardiovascular disease risk factors. Small, statistically non-significant increases in endothelium-dependent flow responses were seen with all treatments. No impairment in response was seen with P4 alone or in combination with E2. The authors concluded that progesterone does not have detrimental vascular effects in humans.*

Molinari C, Battaglia A. Effect of progesterone on peripheral blood flow in prepubertal female anesthetized pigs. *J Vasc Res.* 2001; 38:569-577.

Progesterone dilates coronary arteries by increasing nitric oxide.

Otsuki M, Saito H, Xu X, Sumitani S, Kouhara H, Kishimoto T, Kasayama S. Progesterone, but not medroxyprogesterone, inhibits vascular cell adhesion molecule-1 expression in human vascular endothelial cells. *Arterioscler Thromb Vasc Biol.* 2001 Feb;21(2):243-8.

This study utilizing human umbilical vein endothelial cells (HUVEC's) demonstrated that progesterone, but not medroxyprogesterone acetate (MPA) inhibited expression of vascular cell adhesion molecule-1 (VCAM-1), demonstrating a role for progesterone in the prevention of atherosclerosis. The differing effects of progesterone and MPA are clinically important, as MPA is widely used in hormone replacement therapy, when, as this research suggests, progesterone might be a more appropriate option.*

Rosano GM, Webb CM, Chierchia S, Morgani GL, Gabraele M, Sarrel PM, de Ziegler D, Collins P. Natural Progesterone, but not medroxyprogesterone acetate, enhances the beneficial effect of estrogen on exercise-induced myocardial ischemia in postmenopausal women. *J Am Coll Cardiol.* 2000; 36(7):2154-9.

This randomized crossover study compared the effects of estradiol (E2) (2mg/day), estradiol + Progesterone (P4) vaginal gel (2 mg/day + 90 mg on alternate days), and estradiol + medroxyprogesterone acetate (MPA) (2 mg/day + 10 mg/day) on exercise-induced myocardial ischemia in eighteen postmenopausal women with coronary artery disease (CAD) or previous myocardial infarction (MI). Utilizing treadmill testing, patients were evaluated for exercise tolerance after each estradiol phase and at day 10 of each progestogen phase. The results demonstrated an increase in exercise tolerance with both E2 alone and E2 + progesterone, but not by E2 + MPA as compared to baseline. Furthermore, E2 + P4 demonstrated a significant increase in exercise tolerance when compared to MPA. The results suggest that progesterone may be preferred to progestins for hormone replacement therapy in women at risk for cardiovascular disease.

Rylance PB, Brincat M, Lafferty K, De Trafford JC, Brincat S, Parsons V, Studd JW. Natural progesterone and antihypertensive action. *Br Med J (Clin Res Ed.)* 1985; 290(6461):13-4.

In a placebo controlled, double blind crossover study, increasing doses of natural progesterone were given orally to six men and four postmenopausal women with mild to moderate hypertension who were not receiving any other antihypertensive drugs. Compared to before treatment values and to placebo, progesterone caused a significant reduction in blood pressure, suggesting that progesterone has an antihypertensive action rather than a hypertensive one as has been previously thought. The authors suggest this protective effect of progesterone should be investigated further.

Progesterone
Cortisol

Shmidt M, Renner C, Lofler G. Blocks Cortisol induced expression of aromatase in human adipose tissue. *J Endocrinol.* 1998; 158:401-407.

Progesterone inhibits glucocorticoid-dependent aromatase induction in human adipose fibroblasts.

Progesterone
Cortisol and Sleep

Montplaisir J., Lorrain J., Denesle R. Sleep in menopause: differential effects of two forms of hormone replacement therapy *Menopause.* 2001; 8:10-16.

Progesterone promotes normal sleep patterns, fewer awakenings.

Stephenson, K. et. al. Transdermal progesterone significantly relieves menopausal symptoms in postmenopausal women assessed by Greene Climacteric Scale scores. *Blood* (Annual Meeting Abstracts). 2004 104. Abstract 5318.

Progesterone cream lowered night time cortisol levels.

Progesterone
Brain and Nervous System

Baulieu E, Schumacher M. Progesterone as a neuroactive neurosteroid, with special reference to the effect of progesterone on myelination. *Steroids* 2000; 65(10-11):605-12.

This paper reviews the effects of progesterone on the Brain, with special focus on its role in the formation of the myelin sheath surrounding nerve fibers. Other roles of progesterone in the brain include activating GABA receptors, which induces a calming effect.

Balieu EE, Neurosteroids with special reference to effect of progesterone on myelination peripheral nerves. *Mult Scle. 1997;* 3:105-112.

Progesterone promotes myelin repair.

Frye, C. A., and T. I. Scalise. 2000. Anti-seizure effects of progesterone and 3 alpha, 5 alpha-THP in kainic acid and perforant pathway models of epilepsy. *Psychoneuroendocrinology.* 25:407-420.

Progesterone has an anti-seizure effect.

Gibson CL, Murphy SP. Progesterone enhances functional recovery after middle cerebral artery occlusion in male mice. *J Cereb Blood Flow Metab.* 2004 Jul;24(7):805-13.

Differences in outcomes following ischemia have been noted between men and women, and this is thought to be attributed to sex steroids. This study investigated the potential benefits of progesterone administration after focal cerebral ischemia of the middle cerebral artery of male mice. Male mice undergoing 60-minute middle cerebral artery occlusion (MCAO) received either progesterone or vehicle following occlusion. The mice receiving progesterone had significantly reduced lesion volume (p< 0.05) when compared with the vehicle treated mice (control). Progesterone treatment also improved survival rate, weight recovery, and motor ability when compared to the control group. In addition, mice treated with progesterone demonstrated motor ability comparable to mice that did not undergo MCAO. The authors suggest the need to further investigate the mechanisms of progesterone action on recovery from cerebral injury.

Grossman KJ, Goss CW, Stein DG. Effects of progesterone on the inflammatory response to brain injury in the rat. *Brain Res.* 2004; 1008(1):29-39.

Progesterone has a known anti-inflammatory effect. In this study, male rats treated with progesterone (4 mg/kg) and/or vehicle, were examined with respect to cellular inflammatory response to frontal cortex injury on postsurgical days 1, 3, 5, 7 and 9. The treated mice suffered significantly less edema than untreated mice, as well as showed an increase in the accumulation of activated microglia, demonstrating a neuroprotective effect on the rat brain.

Herzog AG. Progesterone therapy in women with complex partial and secondary generalized seizures. *Neurology* .1995 Sep; 45(9):1660-2.

Progesterone has an anti-seizure effect.

Koenig HL. et. al. *Science* 1995. Jul; 265 (5216): 1500-3.

Progesterone promotes myelin repair.

Koenig HL, Schumacher M, Ferzaz B, Thi AN, Ressouches A, Guennoun R, Jung-Testas I, Robel P, Akwa Y, Baulieu EE. Progesterone synthesis and myelin formation by Schwann cells. *Science.* 1995 Jun 9; 268(5216):1500-3.

Progesterone promotes myelin repair.

Roof RL, Duvdevani R, Stein DG; Gender influences outcome of brain injury: progesterone plays a protective role. *Brain Res.* 1993 Apr 2; 607(1-2):336-6.

Progesterone protects brain following traumatic injury.

Sayeed I, Stein DG. Progesterone as a neuroprotective factor in traumatic and ischemic Brain injury. *Prog Brain Res.* 2009; 175:219-37.

This review describes the effectiveness of progesterone in the treatment of traumatic brain injury, and then focuses on its potential role in the treatment of ischemic stroke. Progesterone and its natural metabolites act through numerous mechanisms to exert their neuroprotective activity, and these are described in the review. The authors recommend testing progesterone in clinical trials as a compelling natural treatment for nervous system injuries such as traumatic brain injury and stroke.*

Schumacher M, Guennoun R, Robert F, Carelli C, Gago N, Ghoumari A, Gonzalez Deniselle MC, Gonzalez SL, Ibanez C, Labombarda F, Coirini H, Baulieu EE, De Nicola AF. Local synthesis and dual actions of progesterone in the nervous system: neuroprotection and myelination. *Growth Horm IGF Res.* 2004; 14 Suppl A:S18-33.

This paper reviews of the effects of progesterone as an autocrine/paracrine hormone in the brain. The brain, spinal cord and peripheral nerves all synthesize progesterone from the precursor, pregnenolone. Macroglial cells, including astrocytes, oligodendroglial cells and Schwann cells, also have the capacity to synthesize progesterone. This production is regulated by cellular interactions.

Recent research has suggested the role progesterone plays in the brain is likely a significant one, supporting the viability of neurons and the formation of myelin sheaths. In mice and rat studies, progesterone also demonstrated a neuroprotective effect. These actions of progesterone suggest viable therapeutic possibilities for the prevention and treatment of neurodegenerative diseases, as well as for repair processes and for preserving cognitive functions with age.

Schumacher M, Guennoun R, Ghoumari A, Massaad C, Robert F, El-Etr M, Akwa Y, Rajkowski K, Baulieu EE. Novel perspectives for progesterone in hormone replacement therapy, with special reference to the nervous system. *Endocr Rev.* 2007; 28(4):387-439.

The authors describe in detail the neuroprotective effects of progesterone when used in postmenopausal hormone replacement therapy. They emphasize that natural progesterone has very different properties than synthetic progestins. Medroxyprogesterone acetate actually inhibits the beneficial effects of estradiol on the nervous system and also exerts damaging effects, whereas progesterone does neither. Progesterone is known to have neuroprotective, neurotrophic, and promyelinating effects.

Schumacher M, Guennoun R, Robert F, Carelli C, Gago N, Ghoumari A, Gonzalez Deniselle MC, Gonzalez SL, Ibanez C, Labombarda F, Coirini H, Baulieu EE, De Nicola AF. Local synthesis and dual actions of progesterone in the nervous system: neuroprotection and myelination. *Growth Horm IGF Res.* 2004; 14 Suppl A:S18-33.

This paper reviews of the effects of progesterone as an autocrine/paracrine hormone in the brain. The brain, spinal cord and peripheral nerves all synthesize progesterone from the precursor, pregnenolone. Macroglial cells, including astrocytes, oligodendroglial cells and Schwann cells, also have the capacity to synthesize progesterone. This production is regulated by cellular interactions. Recent research has suggested the role progesterone plays in the brain is likely a significant one, supporting the viability of neurons and the formation of myelin sheaths. In mice and rat studies, progesterone *also demonstrated a neuroprotective effect. These actions of progesterone suggest viable therapeutic possibilities for the prevention and treatment of neurodegenerative diseases, as well as for repair processes and for preserving cognitive functions with age.*

Schumacher M, Baulieu EE. Neurosteroids: Synthesis and functions in the central and peripheral nervous systems. *Civa Found Symp* 1995; 191:90-106; discussion 106-112.

Progesterone promotes myelin repair.

Sherwin BB. Progestogens used in menopause. Side effects, mood and quality of life. *J Reprod Med.* 1999; 44(2 Suppl):227-32.

This review summarizes the effects of progesterone on mood and other brain functions. Progesterone receptors are present in many of the same areas of the brain as estrogen receptors, including the limbic system and hypothalamus. The limbic system plays a prominent role in regulating mood and emotion. As a comparison, progesterone decreases brain excitability, while estrogens increase it. This relates to why women with epilepsy have a higher frequency of seizures during the part of the cycle when estrogen levels are high, and a reduced frequency when progesterone levels are high. Estrogen and progesterone may also have differing effects on MAO, thereby affecting concentration of serotonin (a mood elevator) in the brain.*

Singh M., Ovarian hormones elicit phosphorylation of Akt and extracellular-signal regulated kinase in explants of the cerebral cortex. *Endocrine.* 2001 Apr;14(3):407-15.

Collectively, the data offer novel mechanisms for both progesterone and estrogen action in the central nervous system, demonstrating the functional and mechanistic diversity of gonadal hormones and supporting their neuroprotective potential for such neurodegenerative disorders as Alzheimer disease.*

Wright DW, Kellermann AL, Hertzberg VS, Clark PL, Frankel M, Goldstein FC, Salomone JP, Dent LL, Harris OA, Ander DS, Lowery DW, Patel MM, Denson DD, Gordon AB, Wald MM, Gupta S, Hoffman SW, Stein DG. ProTECT: a randomized clinical trial of progesterone for acute traumatic brain injury. *Ann Emerg Med.* 2007; 49(4):391-402, 402.e1-2.

A neuroprotective effect of progesterone was observed in this randomized, placebo-controlled trial of very high dose, intravenous progesterone therapy given for 3 days after acute traumatic brain injury. Only 13% of the patients died within 30 days after injury in the progesterone group, compared with 30% of the placebo group, and the progesterone group was more likely to have a moderate to good functional outcome after 30 days than the placebo group. Even at the extremely high dose used, no serious adverse events were seen with progesterone.

Estrogen

Smith, P., *HRT: The Answers.* Traverse City, MI.: Healthy Living Books, 2003; Inc., p. 11.

Sinatra, S., *Heart Sense for Women.* Washington, DC: LifeLine Press, 2000, p. 205.

Estrogen
Heart Disease

Dubey RK, Gillespie DG, Jackson EK, Keller PJ. 17Beta-estradiol, its metabolites, and progesterone inhibit cardiac fibroblast growth. *Hypertension.* 1998 Jan; 31(1 Pt 2):522-8.

Gerhard M, Walsh B, Tawokol A, et al. Estradiol with or without progesterone and ambulatory blood pressure in postmenopausal women. *Hypertension.* 1999 May; 33(5):1190-4.

Ho JY, Chen MJ, Sheu WH, Yi YC, Tsai AC, Guu HF, Ho ES, Differential effects of oral conjugated equine estrogen and transdermal estrogen on atherosclerotic vascular disease risk markers and endothelial function in healthy postmenopausal women. *Hum Reprod.* 2006; 21(10):2715-20.

In this comparison of 0.625 mg/day oral conjugated equine estrogen (CEE) versus 0.6 mg/day 17B-estradiol transdermal gel for 6 months or no treatment, the oral CEE group showed significantly increased levels of C-reactive protein (CRP), a marker of inflammation, while the transdermal and control groups showed no increase in CRP. The transdermal estradiol group showed a similar beneficial effect on flow-mediated vasodilation in the brachial artery to the CEE group, indicating a comparative therapeutic benefit but without increasing the risk of atherosclerosis.*

Lindoff C, Peterson F, Lecander I, Martinsson G, Astedt B. Transdermal estrogen replacement therapy: beneficial effects on hemostatic risk factors for cardiovascular disease. *Maturitas.* 1996; 24(1-2):43-50.

L'Hermite M, Simoncini T, Fuller S, Genazzani AR. Could transdermal estradiol + progesterone be a safer postmenopausal HRT? A review. *Maturitas* 2008;60(3-4):185-201.

This detailed review examines the way different types of hormone replacement therapy (HRT) affect the cardiovascular system, the brain, and the risk of breast cancer. It discusses the research that shows that non-oral estrogens have more favorable cardiovascular effects, such as improved blood pressure control and lower risk of thrombosis. It discusses the benefits of using natural progesterone rather than synthetic progestins in association with estrogens in HRT. Natural progesterone has a beneficial effect on blood vessels and the brain, and confers less or even no risk of breast cancer, compared with synthetic progestins.*

Lokkegaard E, Andreasen AH, Jacobsen RK, Nielsen LH, Agger C, Lidegaard O. Hormone therapy and risk of myocardial infarction: a national register study. *Eur Heart J.* 2008;29(21):2660-8.

This large population study of Danish postmenopausal women found that transdermal estrogen therapy was associated with a significantly lower risk of myocardial infarction than oral unopposed estrogen therapy amongst those using hormone replacement therapy (HRT). The risk of myocardial infarction increased with longer duration of HRT in younger but not older women. A continuous HRT regimen resulted in the greatest risk of myocardial infarction in all age groups, while no increased risk compared to non-HRT users was seen for unopposed estrogen, cyclic estrogen/progestogen HRT, or tibolone. The type of progestogen or dose of estrogen did not appear to affect risk.*

Mendelsohn ME, et al; The Protective Effects of Estrogen on the Cardiovascular System. *NEJM.*1999; June 19, 340(23):1801-1811.

Mosca L; The Role of Hormone Replacement Therapy in the Prevention of Postmenopausal Heart Disease. *Arch Intern Med.* 2000, August 14-28; 160(15):2263-2272.

Ouyang P, Michos ED, Karas RH. Hormone replacement therapy and the cardiovascular system: lessons learned and unanswered questions. *J Am Coll Cardiol* 2006; 47(9):1741-53.

This review discusses the lack of benefit of estrogen therapy in older women for the prevention of cardiovascular problems.

Perera M, Sattar N, Petrie JR, Hillier C, Small M, Connell JM, Lowe GD, Lumsden MA. The effects of transdermal estradiol in combination with oral norethisterone on lipoproteins, coagulation, and endothelial markers in postmenopausal women with Type 2 diabetes: a randomized, placebo-controlled study. *J Clin Endocrinol Metab.* 2001; 86(3):1140-3.

This study showed that transdermal estradiol and oral norethis-
terone reduce plasma triglyceride and total cholesterol levels, factor
VII activity and von Willebrand factor antigen levels in women with
Type 2 diabetes without a concurrent change in adiposity or gly-
cemic control. The authors suggest that this protocol might be of
benefit for women at high risk of cardiovascular disease.*

Pelzer T, et al; Estrogen Effects in the Heart. *Molecular and Cellular*
Biochemistry. 1996; 160/161:307-313.

Snabes MC, et al; Physiologic Estradiol Replacement Therapy and
Cardiac Structure and Function in the Normal Postmenopausal
Women: A Randomized, Double-Blind, Placebo-Controlled, Cross-
over Trial. *Obstetrics & Gynecology.* March 1997, 89(3):332-339.

Zegura B, Keber I, Sebestjen M, Koenig W. Double blind, randomized study of estradiol replacement therapy on markers of
inflammation, coagulation and fibrinolysis. *Atherosclerosis* 2003;
168(1):123-9.

This study on oral and transdermal estradiol found that both
forms of estradiol decreased fibrinogen levels, transdermal estra-
diol did not raise CRP while oral estradiol raised CRP. Both oral
and transdermal estradiol reduced fasting glucose.

Zegura B, Keber I, Sebestjen M, Borko E. Orally and transdermally
replaced estradiol improves endothelial function equally in middle-
aged women after surgical menopause. *Am J Obstet Gynecol* 2003;
188(5):1291-6.

Forty-three surgically induced (6 weeks postop) menopausal
women were randomly assigned in a double-blind study to 28 weeks
of oral or transdermal estradiol. Looking at blood flow through the
brachial artery, flow-mediated dilation (ultrasound) in the oral group
increased 6.0 to 13.2% and in the transdermal group increased 7.0
to 14.9% Results indicate that both oral and transdermal adminis-

tration had equal effect on arterial endothelium independent of lipid profiles and increased vasodilation.*

Estrogen
Bone Building

Arrenbrecht S, Boermans AJ., Effects of transdermal estradiol delivered by a matrix patch on bone density in hysterectomized, postmenopausal women: a 2-year placebo-controlled trial.*Osteoporosis Int.* 2002; 13(2):176-83.

Collette J, Viethel P, Dethor M, Chevallier T, Micheletti MC, Foidart JM, Reginster JY. Comparison of changes in biochemical markers of bone turnover after 6 months of hormone replacement therapy with either transdermal 17 beta-estradiol or conjugated equine estrogen plus nomegestrol acetate. *Gynecol Obstet Fertil.* 2003; 31(5):434-41.

Evans SF, Davie MW. Low and conventional dose transdermal oestradiol are equally effective at preventing bone loss in spine and femur at all post-menopausal ages. *Clin Endocrinol (Oxf).* 1996; 44(1):79-84.

A study compared oral conjugated estrogen and transdermal estradiol per day on biochemical markers of bone resorption in 60 healthy menopausal women. Both therapies were equally effective in that they decreased hydroxyproline/creatine ratios as well as pyridinoline/creatine ratios.

Prestwood KM, Kenny AM, Kleppinger A, Kulldorff M. Ultralowdose micronized 17ß-estradiol and bone density and bone metabolism in older women: a randomized controlled trial. *JAMA.* 2003; 290(8):1042-8.

This study of 0.25 mg/day oral estradiol versus placebo for 3 years in women over 65 years old (with 100 mg/day oral micronized progesterone in women with a uterus in both groups) found an increase in bone density in the estradiol group compared with placebo.*

Prestwood KM, Kenny AM, Unson C, Kulldorff M. The effect of low dose micronized 17beta-estradiol on bone turnover, sex hormone levels, and side effects in older women: a randomized, double blind, placebo-controlled study. *J Clin Endocrinol Metab.* 2000; 85(12):4462-9.

This study determined that oral low-dose estrogen (0.25mg/day) had similar beneficial effects on bone health in elderly (mean age 75 years) postmenopausal women without the breast tenderness and bleeding associated with higher doses. Authors recommended the use of serum E2 levels as the guide for therapeutic effect at a range of 10-28 pg/L.

Reginster JY, Christiansen C, Dequinze B et al. Effect of transdermal 17 beta-estradiol and oral conjugated equine estrogens on biochemical parameters of bone resorption in natural menopause. *Calcified Tissue International.* 1993; 53:13-16.

Estrogen
Brain Function

Bruce-Keller AJ, Keeling JL, Keller JN, Huang FF, Camondola S, Mattson MP. Antiinflammatory effects of estrogen on microglial activation. *Endocrinology.* 2000;141(10):3646-56.

This study identified new pathways for the estrogenic anti-inflammatory effects on brain function, potentially leading to identification of new methods for improving neurodegenerative disease, specifically involving the microglial cells.

Bonnefont AB, Munoz FJ, Inestrosa NC. Estrogen protects neuronal cells from the cytotoxicity induced by acetylcholinesterase-amyloid complexes. *FEBS Lett.* 1998; 441:220-224.

B-amyloid induces an inflammatory response in the brain, which is a large part of the pathologic effect of AD. Some studies have shown that estradiol may inhibit the inflammatory responses by suppressing the homing and activation of inflammatory cells.*

Jacobs, D. et al., Cognitive function in nondeminated older women who took estrogen after menopause. *Neurology* 1998; 50(2):368-373.

Kim H, Bang OY, Jung MW, et al. Neuroprotective effects of estrogen against beta-amyloid toxicity are mediated by estrogen receptors in cultured neuronal cells. *Neurosci Lett* 2001; 302:58-62.

Estrogen appears to enhance the clearance of B-amyloid through microglia, which are key components of the immune system that remove B-amyloid deposits from the brain.

Li R, Shen Y, Yang LB, et al. Estrogen enhances uptake of amyloid beta-protein by microglia derived from the human cortex. *J Neurochem* 2000; 75:1447-1454.

Both B-amyloid and B-amyloid-AchE complexes are ameliorated by estradiol therapy, which provides protection against amyloid-induced toxicity at the cellular level.

Maki PM, et al; Longitudinal Effects of Estrogen Replacement Therapy on PET Cerebral Blood Flow and Cognition. *Neurobiology of Aging.* 2000. 21:373-383.

Shaywitz SE, et al; Effect of Estrogen on Brain Activation Patterns in Postmenopausal Women During Working Memory Tasks. *JAMA.* April 7, 1999 281 (13): 1197-1202.

Birge SJ; Is There a Role for Estrogen Replacement Therapy in the Prevention and Treatment of Dementia? *JAGS.* July 1996; 44(7):865-870.

Shepherd JE, Effects of Estrogen on Cognition, Mood, and Degenerative Brain Diseases. *J. Am Pharm Assoc.* 2001; 41:221-228.

Sherwin BB; Can Estrogen Keep You Smart? Evidence from Clinical Studies. *J Psychiatry Neuroscience.* Sep 2, 1999; 24(4):315-321.

Sherwin BB; Estrogen Effects in Cognition in Menopausal Women. *Neurology.* 1997; 4(supple7):S21-S26.

Sherwin BB; Estrogenic Effects on Memory in Women. *Depts. Psychology, Obstetrics & Gynecology.* McGill Univ. pp. 213-231.

Sherwin BB; Oestrogen and Cognitive Function Throughout the Female Lifespan. *Depts. Psychology, Obstets & Gynecology,* McGill University. Pp. 188-201.

Warga, Claire,. *Menopause and the Mind.* The Free Press, New York, NY. 1999.

Estrogen
Depression

Cohen LS, Soares CN, Poitras JR, Prouty J, Alexander AB, Shifren JL. Short-term use of estradiol for depression in perimenopausal and postmenopausal women: a preliminary report. *Am J Psychiatry.* 2003; 160(8):1519-22.

Twenty-two peri- or post-menopausal women with median age of 50 years experiencing moderate severity depression (DSM-IV major depression, minor depression, or dysthymia) were enrolled in a 4 week open-label clinical trial of 100 micrograms of transdermal 17B estradiol. Results showed decreased score on Montgomery-Asberg Depression Rating Scale (20 to 11.50) and Beck Depression Inventory. Greene-Climacteric Scale scores showed measured improvement during the 4 week study. Changes in depression scales and climacteric scales were not significantly correlated. Perimenopausal (6) women showed greater improvement in depression scales than *postmenopausal women (2). Authors suggested this study supports previous results showing that the effect of estrogen therapy on mood may be independent of antidepressant effects mediated by alleviation of vasomotor symptoms and that estrogen therapy may be of benefit to perimenopausal women experiencing moderately severe depression.**

Estrogen
Hot Flashes and Menopausal Symptoms

Archer DF, Estrogel Study Group., Percutaneous 17beta-estradiol gel for the treatment of vasomotor symptoms in postmenopausal women. *Menopause.* 2003; 10(6):516-21.

The frequency of moderate-to-severe hot flashes was significantly reduced after once daily application of estradiol gel for 12 weeks, compared to placebo gel, in 221 postmenopausal women. Two doses of estradiol gel were used: 1.25 g, containing 0.75 mg estradiol, and 2.5 g, containing 1.5 mg estradiol. Both were effective and well tolerated, although the higher dose resulted in more estrogen-related adverse events.*

Wepfer ST., Part 1 - The science behind bioidentical hormone replacement therapy. *Int J Pharm Compounding.* 2001; 5(6):10-12.

The author defines bioidentical hormone therapy and reviews the scientific literature supporting its use to treat menopausal symptoms, focusing on the 3 Estrogens: estrone, estradiol, and estriol, as well as progesterone and testosterone.*

Safety of Bioidentical Estradiol

Jarupanich T, Lamlertkittikul S, Chandeying V., Efficacy, safety and acceptability of a seven-day, transdermal estradiol patch for estrogen replacement therapy. *J Med Assoc Thai* 2003;86(9):836-45.

Estrogen
Weight and Metabolism

Asarian L et al., Bioidentical estradiol increases CCK, satiety, and decreases food intake. *Philos Trans R Soc Lond B Biol Sci.* 2006 Jul 29; 361(1471):1251-63.

Edler C et al., Decline of estrogen leads to binge-eating. *Psychol Med.* 2006 Oct 12;:1-11.

Gao H et al.,Prolonged estradiol treatment increases insulin sensitivity. *Mol Endocrinol.* 2006 Jun;20(6):1287-99.

Klopfenstein BJ, Samuels MH, Purnell JQ. Oregon Health & Science University, Portland, Oregon Estrogen therapy reduces 24-hour free cortisol levels in postmenopausal women. Abstract of research presented at Endocrine Society annual meeting, Summer, 2005.

Estrogen maybe effective as a treatment to reduce obesity in post-menopausal women.

Klopfenstein BJ. Oregon Health & Science University, Portland, Oregon, 24-hour Cortisol Production Rates, Free Cortisol, and Intra-Abdominal Fat Are Elevated in Postmenopausal Women but Are Similar in Premenopausal and Postmenopausal Women Taking Hormone Replacement Therapy. Abstract of research presented at Endocrine Society annual meeting Summer, 2003.

Estrogen may be effective as a treatment to reduce obesity in post-menopausal women.

Micheline,CC., et al. ,Bioidentical estradiol applied to skin decreases ghrelin. *Fertil Steril.* 2006 Dec;86(6)1669.

http://www.ohsu.edu/ohsuedu/newspub/releases/menopausal060605.cfm?WT_rank=1

Oregon Health & Science University researchers unveiled research results that help explain why middle-aged women develop central body fat. The announcement will take place during the 2005 Society for Endocrinology annual meeting today in San Diego. The OHSU research team has also conducted initial testing of estrogen replacement therapy as a possible method for counteracting the problem.

Estriol

Estriol
Breasts or Breast Cancer

AB D'Assoro, R Busby, ID Acu, C Quatraro, MM Reinholz, DJ Farrugia, MA Schroeder, C Allen, F Stivala, E Galanis, and JL Salisbury., Impaired p53 function leads to centrosome amplification, acquired ERα phenotypic heterogeneity and distant metastases in breast cancer MCF-7 xenografts. *Oncogene.* 2005 Oct 6; 24(44):6605-16.

Hartman J et al. Estriol prevents breast cancer cells from producing new blood vessels and VEGF: *Cancer Res.* 2006 Dec 1;66(23):11207-13.

Kuiper GG, Enmark E, Pelto-Huikko M, Nilsson S, Gustafsson JA. Cloning of a novel receptor expressed in rat prostate and ovary. *Proc Natl Acad Sci U S A.* 1996 Jun 11;93(12):5925-30.

Lemon HM; Kumar PF; Peterson C; Rodriguez-Sierra JF; Abbo KM Inhibition of radiogenic mammary carcinoma in rats by estriol or tamoxifen. *Cancer* 1989 May 1;63(9):1685-92.

Lemon HM; Wotiz HH; Parsons L; Mozden PJ Reduced estriol excretion in patients with breast cancer prior to endocrine therapy. *JAMA* 1966 Jun 27;196(13):1128-36.

Lemon, H.M. Pathophysiologic considerations in the treatment of menopausal patients with oestrogens; the role of oestriol in the prevention of mammary carcinoma. *Acta Endocrinol Suppl* 1980 233:17-27. DNH.

Melamed M, Castano E, Notides A, Sasson S. Molecular and kinetic basis for the mixed agonist/antagonist activity of estriol. *Mol Endocrinology.* Nov 1997; 11(12):1868-78.

Paech K, Webb P, Kuiper GG, Nilsson S, Gustafsson J, Kushner PJ, Scanlan TS. Differential ligand activation of estrogen receptors ERalpha and ERbeta at AP1 sites. *Science.* 1997 Sep 5; 277(5331):1508-10.

Paruthiyil S, Parmar H, Kerekatte V, Cunha GR, Firestone GL, Leitman DC. Estrogen receptor beta inhibits human breast cancer cell proliferation and tumor formation by causing a G2 cell cycle arrest. *Cancer Res.* 2004 Jan 1; 64(1):423-8.

Shah, N., Wong, T. Current breast cancer risks of hormone replacement therapy in postmenopausal women. *Int J Cancer.* 1999 May 5; 81(3):339-44.

Sitieri PK, Sholtz PI, Cirillo PM, et al. Prospective study of estrogens during pregnancy and the risk of breast cancer. Unpublished study performed at the Public Health Institute in Oakland, California, and funded by the US Army Medical Research and Material Command under DAMD 17- 99-1-9358.

This 35 year study showed a significant protective role of estriol against breast cancer.

Wright JV. Bio-identical steroid hormone replacement: selected observations from 23 years of clinical and laboratory practice. *Ann N Y Acad Sci.* 2005;1057:506-24.

This review discusses the types of Estrogens used in bioidentical hormone replacement, including their dosages and routes of administration. The author advocates the use of natural hormones because of the problems with using non-human identical synthetic hormones, highlighted largely by the Women's Health Initiative trial. However, bioidentical estrogens must be properly monitored to ensure appropriate dosing, just as is common for thyroid hormone replacement. The metabolism of estradiol to estrone and estriol is discussed. The author advocates the use of iodine supplements, which stimulate the metabolism of estradiol towards estriol. The amount of circulating estriol relative to estradiol and estrone is important in breast cancer risk: the greater the relative amount of estriol, the lower the breast cancer risk.*

Zhu BT et al., Quantitative structure-activity relationship of various endogenous estrogen metabolites for human estrogen receptor alpha and beta subtypes: Insights into the structural determinants favoring a differential subtype binding. *Endocrinology.* 2007; 148(2):538-547.

Estriol affects beta receptors that decrease breast tissue proliferation.

Zhu BT et al.,Virtual screening of the estrogen receptor. *Endocrinology.*2006 Sep;147(9):4132-50.

Estriol affects beta receptors that decrease breast tissue proliferation.

Estriol
Treatment of Menopausal Symptoms

Lauritzen C. Results of a 5 years prospective study of estriol succinate treatment in patients with climacteric complaints. *Horm Metab Res.* 1987 Nov;19(11):579-84.

Paoletti J. The physiologic role and use of estriol. *Int J Pharm Compounding* 2009;13(4)270-275.

Estriol has an important physiological role in the prevention of breast cancer by balancing the effects of the stronger estrogens, estradiol and estrone, effectively acting as an anti-estrogen. The author explains this phenomenon and explains a rationale for appropriate dosing of estriol relative to estradiol in bioidentical hormone replacement therapy.*

Takahashi K, Manabe A, Okada M, Kurioka H, Kanasaki H, Miyazaki K., Efficacy and safety of oral estriol for managing postmenopausal symptoms. *Maturitas* 2000;34(2):169-77.

Takahashi K, Okada M, Ozaki T, Kurioka H, Manabe A, Kanasaki H, Miyazaki K. Safety and efficacy of oestriol for symptoms of natural or surgically induced menopause. *Hum Reprod* 2000;15(5):1028-36.

The authors gave 2 mg/day oral estriol for one year to 53 postmenopausal women (aged 40-62). None of the patients stopped treatment due to side effects; level of satisfaction with the treatment increased throughout the study, and averaged at 85% in naturally menopausal women and 93% in surgically menopausal women by the end of the year. Menopausal symptoms were significantly reduced. No distinctive effects on bone or lipid levels were seen. The authors suggest that estriol is a good choice of HRT to reduce symptoms in women who are not susceptible to osteoporosis or coronary artery disease.*

Tzingounis VA; Aksu MF; Greenblatt RB Estriol in the management of the menopause *JAMA* 1978 Apr 21;239(16):1638-41.

Yang TS et al.; *Maturitas.* Efficacy and safety of estriol replacement therapy for climacteric women. 2000 Feb 15;34(2):169-77.

Yang TS, Tsan SH, Chang SP, Ng HT. Estriol quickly alleviates night sweats and hot flashes. *JAMA.* 1978 Apr 21;239(16):1638-41.

Estriol
Endometrium and Ovaries

Granberg S, Eurenius K, Lindgren R, Wilhelmsson L., The effects of oral estriol on the endometrium in postmenopausal women. *Maturitas* 2002;42(2):149-56.

This study conducted endometrial evaluation using both transvaginal ultrasound (TVS) and histologic biopsy by Pipelle in postmenopausal women taking a low-dose oral estriol (1 or 2 mg daily) for a mean duration of 4.3 years. Mean endothelial thickness in the study group after one year was 3.0mm and in the control group was 2.4mm. There was a noted increase in atrophic vaginal epithelium in the control group. There was a noted increased incidence of endometrial polyps in the study group (14.1%) compared to the control group (2.9%) although this was not determined to be clinically significant.

Weiderpass E, Baron JA, Adami HO, Magnusson C, Lindgren A, Bergstrom R, Correia N, Persson I. Low-potency estrogen and risk of endometrial cancer: a case-control study. *Lancet.* 1999 May 29;353(9167):1824-8.

Estriol and Endometrial Cancer Risk 1999: This study showed that when given by the proper "route of administration" (always transdermal, never oral) estriol does not increase risk of endometrial cancer.

Treeck O et al.Estriol has anti tumor effect on ovarian cancer cell: *J Endo Crinol.* 2007 Jun;193(3):421-33.

Estriol
Bone Density or Cardiovascular Function

Hayashi T, Ito I, Kano H, Endo H, Iguchi A. Estriol (E3) replacement improves endothelial function and bone mineral density in very elderly women. *J Gerontol A Biol Sci Med Sci.* 2000 Apr;55(4):B183-90; discussion B191-3.

This study showed that estriol treatment improved bone density and reduced atherosclerosis parameters in elderly females.

Kano H, Hayashi T, Sumi D, Matusi-Hirai H, Tsunekawa T, Endo H, Iguchi A. Estriol retards and stabilizes atherosclerosis through an NO-mediated system. *Life Sci.* 2002 May 24;71(1):31-42.

Estriol, Atherosclerosis and Nitric Oxide: This study shows that estriol has anti-atherosclerotic effects.

Minaguchi H, Uemura T, Shirasu K, et al. Effect of estriol on bone loss in postmenopausal Japanese women: a multicenter prospective open study. J *Obstet Gynaecol Res.* 1996 Jun;22(3):259-65.

Nishibe A, Morimoto S, Hirota K, et al. Effect of estriol and bone mineral density of lumbar vertebrae in elderly and postmenopausal women. *Nippon Ronen Igakkai Zasshi.* 1996 May;33(5):353-9.

Mishra RG et. Al, *Am J Physiol Heart Circ Physiol.* 2006 Jan;290(1):H295-303.

Yamanaka Y et al., *Gynecol Endocrinol.* 2003 Dec;17(6):455-61.

Estriol
Safety

Head KA., Estriol: safety and efficacy. *Altern Med Rev* 1998;3(2):101-13.

The author reviews research on estriol, particularly looking at its effectiveness in treating menopausal symptoms, and in protecting against osteoporosis and cardiovascular disease. Estriol is a weaker estrogen than estradiol or estrone, and has been found to be effective in controlling symmptoms such as hot flashes, insomnia, *vaginal dryness, and frequent urinary tract infections. Estriol was not shown to effectively prevent bone loss except in some Japanese studies, and the author speculates that the Japanese diet with its phytoestrogen content may have been a factor. Estriol's protective effect against cardiovascular disease has not been well studied.**

Estriol
Urinary Track Infections and Vaginal Health

Dessole S, Rubattu G, Ambrosini G et al. Efficacy of low-dose intravaginal estriol on urogenital aging in postmenopausal women. *Menopause.* 2004 Jan; 11(1):49-56.

Iosif, CS., Department of Obstetrics and Gynecology, University of Lund, Sweden.

Effects of Protracted Administration of Estriol on the Lower Genito Urinary Tract in Post-Menopausal Women. *Arch Ghyecol Obstet* 1992;251(3):115-20.

Lose G, Englev E. Department of Obstetrics and Gynaecology, Glostrup County Hospital, Copenhagen University, Denmark. Oestradiol-Releasing Vaginal Ring Versus Oestriol Vaginal Pessaries in the Treatment of Bothersome Lower Urinary Tract Symptoms. Clinical Trial. *BJOG* 2000 Aug; 107(8):1029-34.

Manonai J, Theppisai U. Effect of oral estriol on urogenital symptoms, vaginal cytology, and plasma hormone level in postmenopausal women. *J Med Assoc Thai* 2001;84(4):539-44.

Raz R, Stamm WE.. A controlled trial of intravaginal estriol in postmenopausal women with recurrent urinary tract infections. *N Engl J Med* 1993; 329(11):753-6.

This randomized, double blind, placebo-controlled trial looked at the incidence of urinary tract infections (UTI) in 93 postmenopausal women using 0.5 mg estriol vaginal cream once nightly for *two weeks followed by twice weekly application or placebo. Results showed significantly lower UTI rates in treatment group (0.5 infections per patient-year vs. 5.9 for placebo group). The mean vaginal pH fell from 5.5+-0.7 to 3.6+-1.0 for treatment group and 5.8+-1/2 to 6.1+-2.0 in placebo group and there was an increase in vaginal colonization with lactobacilli in the treatment group. Authors recommend use of topical vaginal estriol in preventive treatment of women with frequent UTI as possible replacement for long-term use of nitrofurantoin, co-trioxazole, trimethoprim, cehpalexin or fluoroquinolones.**

Tzingounis VA et al.Estriol does not promote uterine tissue growth which may decrease the incidence of uterine cancer: *Comp Biochem Physiol C.* 1990;96(2):241-4. Tamaya T et al.; *JAMA.* 1978 Apr 21;239(16):1638-41.

Yoshimura T, Okamura H. Short term oral estriol treatment restores normal premenopausal vaginal flora to elderly women. *Maturitas.* 200; 39(3):253-7.

This study looked at short term (14 days) oral estriol (2.0mg/day) treatment for atrophic vaginitis in 59 postmenopausal women aged 50-75 years. The results showed that in the majority of women in the study group the oral estriol restored normal vaginal flora by the end of the treatment period.

Estriol
Wrinkles

Kainz C, Gitsch G, Stani J, Breitenecker G, Binder M, Schmidt JB. 2nd Department of Gynecology and Obstetrics, University of Vienna, School of Medicine, Austria. When Applied to Facial Skin, Does Estrogen Ointment Have Systemic Effects? *Arch Gynecol Obstet* 1993;253(2):71-4.

Schmidt JB, et al.; Treatment of Skin Aging with Topical Estrogens. *Int J Dermatol.* 1996 Sept; 35(9):669-674.

Estriol
Multiple Sclerosis

Soldan SS, varez Retuerto AI, Sicotte NL, Voskuhl RR. Immune modulation in multiple sclerosis patients treated with the pregnancy hormone estriol. *J Immunol.* 2003 Dec 1;171(11):6267-74.

Estriol
Legal Issues

Goodrum J., Estriol: women's choice vs. a manufacturer's greed. *Int J Pharm Compounding* 2008;12(4):286-292.

This is a response to the FDA's attempt to halt the compounding of hormone preparations containing estriol. The author explains the background to this, which was primarily instigated by the pharmaceutical company Wyeth (manufacturer of Prempro). Estriol has been used clinically for decades without adverse effects when dosed appropriately, and is widely available in Europe. An explanation of actions being taken by the International Association of Compounding Pharmacists to reverse the FDA's ban is given. *

Testosterone

Testosterone
Deficiency and Decline

Burger HG et al. Women's testosterone expression peaks in early 20s and decreases nearly 50% by mid-forties. *Sex Health.* 2006 May;3(2):73-8.

Thorneycroft IH et al.; Oral contraceptives decrease close to 80% of the available testosterone: *Contraception.* 1999 Nov;60(5):255-62.

Rohr UD., Women lose 70% of testosterone within 72 hours after removal of their ovaries: *Maturitas.* 2002 Apr 15;41.

Testosterone
Sexual Benefits

Davis SR., Testosterone for low libido in postmenopausal women not using systemic oestrogen therapy. *Med J Aust.* 2009; 191(3):134-5.

This editorial, written by the principal investigator for the "Aphrodite" study, concludes that the use of transdermal testosterone for hypoactive sexual desire disorder (HSDD) shows promising results but long-term safety requires further study. The article describes the Aphrodite study, in which 814 women with HSDD were randomized to receive a patch delivering 150 or 300 mcg/day testosterone, or placebo patches, for 52 weeks. The testosterone groups reported significantly more satisfying sexual events and reduction of distress, although the frequency of sexual activity did not increase. Benefits were seen after 8 weeks of therapy. No significant adverse effects were seen.*

Krapf JM, Simon JA., The role of testosterone in the management of hypoactive sexual desire disorder in postmenopausal women. *Maturitas.* 2009; 63(3):213-9.

This article reviews testosterone's role in sexual function in women. Research is going on to study the safety and effectiveness of transdermal testosterone therapy in women with low sexual desire, sometimes called HSDD (hypoactive sexual desire disorder) if it leads to distress. The prevalence of this disorder is highest in women who are surgically menopausal, i.e., they have had both ovaries removed, which results in a sudden decline in testosterone levels that leads to a reduced desire for sex and less satisfying sex. The authors review clinical studies of transdermal testosterone therapy, both with and without estrogen, concluding that it is safe and effective in women struggling with HSDD.*

Testosterone
Mood

Hermans EJ et al.,Testosterone significantly reduced women's fear response. *Biol Psychiatry.* 2006 May 1;59(9):872-4.

Nagata H et al., Estrogen improves depression and sexual response. *J Obstet Gynaecol* Res. 2005 Apr;31(2):107-14.

Studd J et al., Testosterone supplementation has positive affect on depression. *Climacteric.*2004 Dec;7(4):338-46.

Testosterone
Bone Density

Flöter A, Nathorst-Böös J, Carlström K, Ohlsson C, Ringertz H, Schoultz B.Effects of combined estrogen/testosterone therapy on bone and body composition in oophorectomized women. *Gynecol Endocrinol.* 2005 Mar;20(3):155-60.

Raisz LG, Wiita B, Artis A, Bowen A, Schwartz S, Trahiotis M, Shoukri K, Smith J. Comparison of the effects of estrogen alone and estrogen plus androgen on biochemical markers of bone formation and resorption in postmenopausal women. *J Clin Endocrinol Metab.* 1996 Jan;81(1):37-43

Tok EC, Ertunc D, Oz U, Camdeviren H, Ozdemir G, Dilek S.The effect of circulating androgens on bone mineral density in post-menopausal women. *Maturitas.* 2004 Jul 15;48(3):235-42.

Turner A, Chen TC, Barber TW, Malabanan AO, Holick MF, Tangpricha V. Testosterone increases bone mineral density in female-to-male transsexuals: a case series of 15 subjects. *Clin Endocrinol (Oxf).* 2004 Nov;61(5):560-6.

Savvas M, Studd JW, Norman S, Leather AT, Garnett TJ, Fogelman I. Increase in bone mass after one year of percutaneous oestradiol and testosterone implants in post-menopausal women who have previously received long-term oral oestrogens. *Br J Obstet Gynaecol.* 1992 Sep;99(9):757-60.

Testosterone
Cardiovascular Disease

Bernini GP et al., Decreased testosterone in menopause increases thickness of carotid artery wall. *J Clin Endocrinol Metab.* 1999 Jun; 84(6):2008-12.

Debing E et al., Decreased testosterone associated with increase atherosclerosis. *Eur J Endocrinol* 2007 Jun; 156(6):689-93.

Montalcini T et al., Decreased testosterone levels associated with increase cardiovascular disease in menopause. *Coron Artery Dis.* 2007 Feb; 18(1):9-13.

Testosterone
Insulin

Svartberg J., Testosterone treatment helpful in preventing and treating diabetes. *Int J Impot Res.* 2006 Jul 20.

Testosterone
Breast Cancer

Hofling M, Hirschberg AL, Skoog L, Tani E, Hägerström T, von Schoultz B.

Testosterone inhibits estrogen/progestogen-induced breast cell proliferation in postmenopausal women. *Menopause.* 2007 Mar-Apr;14(2):183-90.

Labrie F, Luu-The V, Labrie C, Bélanger A, Simard J, Lin SX, Pelletier G. Endocrine and intracrine sources of androgens in women: inhibition of breast cancer and other roles of androgens and their precursor dehydroepiandrosterone. *Endocr Rev.* 2003 Apr;24(2):152-82.

Macedo LF, Guo Z, Tilghman SL, Sabnis GJ, Qiu Y, Brodie A. Role of androgens on MCF-7 breast cancer cell growth and on the inhibitory effect of letrozole.*Cancer Res.* 2006 Aug 1;66(15):7775-82.

Testosterone
Reproductive Function

Massin N. et al., Testosterone supports follicle function. *Hum Reprod.* 2006 May;21(5):1204-11.

CHAPTER 4

Saliva Testing

Summaries provided compliments of ZRT Laboratory in Beaverton, OR. www.zrtlab.com

Aardal E, Holm AC. Cortisol in saliva-reference ranges and relation to cortisol in serum. *Eur J Clin Chem Clin Biochem* 1995;33:927-932.

Parallel serum and saliva samples were acquired in 197 individuals, in the morning and evening. A slight decrease in morning cortisol was seen in the oldest individuals tested (61-70 years). As has been demonstrated in other work, once serum cortisol exceeded 450 nmol/l, a marked increase in salivary cortisol was noted. This is attributed to a rapid increase in free plasma cortisol once the available sites on cortisol binding globulin are filled. The authors conclude by enumerating the advantages of saliva over serum (simplicity, decreased stress, convenience, sample mail-in, temperature stability).

Aardal-Eriksson E, Karlberg BE, Holm AC. Salivary cortisol- an alternative to serum cortisol determinations in dynamic function tests. *Clin Chem Lab Med* 1998;36:215-222.

Serum and salivary cortisol responses were compared in various dynamic tests of HPA axis function including insulin tolerance, CRH stimulation, and ACTH challenge. In 42 of 45 tests performed, consideration of salivary cortisol led to the same conclusion as serum cortisol. The authors conclude that due to a more pronounced cortisol response in saliva, and a closer correlation between salivary cortisol and serum ACTH, salivary cortisol may be used as an alternative parameter in dynamic endocrine tests.

Belkien LD, Bordt J, Moller P, Hano R, Nieschlag E. Estradiol in saliva for monitoring follicular stimulation in an in vitro fertilization program. *Fertil Steril* 1985;44:322.

Serial serum and saliva measurements were compared in 23 patients undergoing ovulation induction in an in vitro fertilization program. Serum and saliva were well correlated (r=0.77) throughout, except for salivary estradiol levels less than 4 pg/ml. (Note that estradiol can easily be detected below this level with modern methods.) The authors conclude that, "assessment of ovarian function in clomiphene citrate (CC) or CC/hMG stimulated cycles can be performed precisely with the saliva estradiol assay."

Bolaji II, Tallon DF, O'Dwyer E, Fottrell PF. Assessment of bioavailability of oral micronized progesterone using a salivary progesterone enzymeimmunoassay. *Gynecol Endocrinol* 1993;7:101-110.

These authors looked at salivary progesterone levels in 40 postmenopausal women taking 100 mg oral micronized progesterone in cyclical fashion (23 days/month) for one year. These levels fell into the range observed in the luteal phases of a control group of 40 normally cycling women. Five patients had simultaneous serum and saliva levels of progesterone measured for 12 hours after ingestion of a 100 mg dose of progesterone. Levels in both cases followed the same time curve, with both peaking at 2 hours. This supports the notion that progesterone diffuses rapidly from serum to saliva.

Campbell BC, Ellison PT. Menstrual variation in salivary testosterone among regularly cycling women. *Horm Res* 1992;37:132-136.

Daily first morning saliva samples were collected from 20 regularly cycling women over the course of an entire menstrual cycle and assayed for testosterone and progesterone. Cycles were classified as ovulatory if salivary progesterone exceeded 100 pg/ml on any day in the cycle. Average testosterone level was significantly greater in anovulatory cycles. In both types of cycle, the same general features were observed: a luteal trough, a midcycle peak, and an early follicular peak, although in non-ovulatory cycles, the midcycle peak was longer, and the luteal trough shorter. These findings are consistent with what is known about changes in ovarian steroid metabolism throughout the menstrual cycle. Salivary assay is particularly well-suited to studies of this nature, which involve multiple measurements, since samples can be acquired with minimal inconvenience.

Choe JK, Khan-Dawood FS, Dawood MY. Progesterone and estradiol in the saliva and plasma during the menstrual cycle. *Am J Obstet Gynecol* 1983;147:557-562.

Daily saliva and blood samples were obtained from 9 women throughout an entire menstrual cycle. Saliva and plasma levels of progesterone correlated reasonably well (r=0.58) although the saliva and blood samples were not acquired at the same time. The percentage of protein binding of progesterone in serum and saliva was also measured by equilibrium dialysis. Forty to fifty percent of the progesterone in saliva was protein bound, compared to three to six percent in plasma. However, unbound progesterone levels in plasma and saliva were comparable, supporting the contention that salivary progesterone represents unbound progesterone in the blood.

The authors also measured salivary and plasma estradiol but did not display or mention the plasma data, commenting only that there was no correlation between levels in the two matrices. This casts suspicion on the validity of their plasma estradiol data.

Clements AD, Parker CR. The relationship between salivary cortisol concentrations in frozen versus mailed samples. *Psychoneuroendocrinol* 1998;23:613-616.

Saliva specimens were obtained from 17 volunteers. Half of each specimen was immediately frozen. The other half was subjected to varying temperatures and physical handling intended to mimic conditions experienced during mailing. Both sample halves were ultimately assayed for cortisol, and a correlation coefficient of 0.92 was derived between the quick-frozen and "mailed" specimens. The authors conclude that mailing saliva samples intended for cortisol assay is acceptable.

Dabbs JM. Salivary testosterone measurements: collecting, storing and mailing saliva samples. *Phys Behav* 1991;49:815-817.

The authors assessed the effect of saliva storage time and storage temperature, the use of stimulants to collect saliva, as well as the effect of cotton swabs for sample collection in salivary testosterone assays. Cotton swabs were found to contribute an apparent testosterone concentration ranging from 20 to 70 pg/ml. Sugar-containing gums elevated apparent testosterone levels by 30 pg/ml. Saliva samples could be stored unrefrigerated for up to 1 week with no effect on apparent testosterone level (specimens from women experienced an increase in apparent testosterone concentration if stored for more than a week at room temperature). The effect of storage time and temperature on apparent testosterone concentration was only studied on 2 men and 2 women, however. The authors conclude, "Salivary measurements provide a robust indicator of subjects' testosterone levels."

Dabbs JM. Salivary testosterone measurements: reliability across hours, days and weeks. *Phys Behav* 1990;48:83-86.

In this study, correlations between sequential measurements of salivary testosterone in men and women across intervals of hours, 2 days, 2 weeks, 5 weeks and 9 weeks were studied. The expected circadian variation, with highest levels in the a.m. was observed. Not surprisingly, correlations between measurements taken weeks apart were only modest, and worsened as the sampling interval increased. Random salivary testosterone levels were obtained from 126 cycling women and plotted as a function of time since last menstruation. No tendency toward a midcycle peak was observed, leading the authors to conclude that in behavioral studies, saliva samples could be acquired without regard to timing in the menstrual cycle.

Dabbs JM, Campbell BC, Gladue BA, Midgley AR, Navarro MA, Read GF, Susman EJ, Swinkels LM, Worthman CM. Reliability of salivary testosterone measurements: a multicenter evaluation. *Clin Chem* 1995;41:1581-1584.

Results of a multicenter evaluation (8 University laboratories, 1 commercial laboratory) of the reliability of salivary testosterone assay are presented in this paper. Each laboratory assayed aliquots of saliva specimens collected from 100 male and 100 female subjects. The intraclass correlation coefficient, which measures overall agreement on individual scores was r=0.87 for men and r=0.78 for women, Mean agreement between each laboratory and the combined set of all other laboratories was r=0.6 (both sexes). The authors concluded that the level of expertise in immunoassay of saliva was gradually increasing.

Granger DA, Schwartz EB, Booth A, Curran M, Zakaria D. Assessing dehydroepiandrosterone in saliva: a simple radioimmunoassay for use in studies of children, adolescents and adults. *Psychoneuroendocrinology* 1999;24:567-579.

Performance of a radioimmunoassay for DHEA in saliva is reported. The authors note, "Levels in matched serum and saliva samples showed strong linear relationships for adult males and females". Reference ranges are provided for children, adolescents and adults. Use of cotton swabs or sugared drinks to aid sample collection resulted in 50-150% overestimation of DHEA content. Failure to extract and preconcentrate specimens likely contributed to the susceptibility of this assay to outside factors.

Harris B, Lovett L, Newcombe RG, Read GF, Walker R, Riad-Fahmy D. Maternity blues and major endocrine changes:Cardiff puerperal mood and hormone study II. *BMJ* 1994 Apr;308:949-953.

These authors studied the relationship of salivary progesterone and cortisol to mood in postpartum women. Salivary progesterone levels peaked just before delivery at roughly 1100 pg/ml, falling to 30 pg/ml by 10 days postpartum. Evening salivary cortisol levels peaked at delivery at around 2400 pg/ml, falling to approximately 600 pg/ml by 15 days postpartum. There were modest, statistically significant correlations between self-rated postpartum depressive symptoms, immediate antepartum progesterone levels and also the rate at which salivary progesterone increased in the 2 weeks preceding delivery. Interestingly, no correlation between postpartum blues and total plasma progesterone (or changes thereof) was seen, demonstrating the utility of saliva as a vehicle to measure clinically significant parameters.

Heine RP, McGregor JA, Dullien VK. Accuracy of salivary estriol testing compared to traditional risk factor assessment in predicting preterm birth. *Am J Obstet Gynecol* 1999;180:S214-218.

Baseline risk of preterm labor was assessed in 601 pregnant women at 21-25 weeks gestation via conventional multifactorial risk assessment (Creasy score). Weekly salivary estriol assays were performed until delivery, and were deemed positive if the result exceeded a threshold of 2100 pg/ml. Salivary estriol screening correctly predicted preterm birth in 91% of cases versus 75% with

Creasy scoring. In patients deemed high risk at baseline, saliva estriol screening was vastly superior, correctly predicting outcome in 87% of cases versus only 7% using Creasy scoring.

Khan-Dawood FS, Choe JK, Dawood MY. Salivary and plasma bound and "free" testosterone in men and women. *Am J Obstet Gynecol* 1984;148:441-445.

Testosterone was measured in matched saliva and plasma samples in a group of men and women. Correlation coefficient for salivary on plasma testosterone was r=0.71. Diurnal variation of testosterone levels was exhibited. Hourly variation of measured values was on the order of 10-15%. On average, dialyzable testosterone in saliva was approximately 60% of that measured in plasma. The authors conclude, "The present investigation showed that salivary testosterone correlates significantly with plasma testosterone and reflects the response of the latter to some of the physiologic variables examined."

Lachelin GC, McGarrigle HH. A comparison of saliva, plasma unconjugated and plasma total oestriol levels throughout normal pregnancy. *Brit J Obstet Gyn* 1984;91:1203-1209.

Parallel plasma and salivary estriol levels were measured weekly in 25 women throughout their second and third trimesters of pregnancy. Levels increased throughout pregnancy and correlation coefficients between results in the two matrices were in excess of 0.9. The percentage of protein binding of unconjugated estriol in plasma was measured by equilibrium dialysis and found to be roughly 12%. This allowed comparison of salivary estriol to free estriol in plasma. Salivary estriol ranged from 85% (early pregnancy) to 120% (late pregnancy) of the plasma free estriol. Hence, salivary estriol levels are very similar, but not identical to free estriol levels in plasma. The authors conclude that, "salivary estriol concentrations parallel those of plasma unconjugated estriol throughout pregnancy and could probably replace them in the assessment of fetal wellbeing."

Lechner W, Marth C, Daxenbichler G. Correlation of oestriol levels in saliva, plasma and urine of pregnant women. *Acta Endocrinol* 1985;109:266-268.

The authors measured conjugated and unconjugated estriol in plasma, urine and saliva in 50 women in their last trimester of pregnancy. They reported significant correlations between unconjugated salivary and total plasma estriol, and between unconjugated plasma and total urinary estriol, but only weak correlation between saliva and urinary estriol. They concluded that no definite conclusion could be drawn regarding the biological significance and clinical importance of salivary estriol.

Lipson SF, Ellison PT. Development of protocols for the application of salivary steroid analyses to field conditions. *Am J Human Biol* 1989;1:249-255.

Practical parameters of interest for the performance of salivary hormone assays (testosterone, progesterone, androstenedione and cortisol) were examined in this study. Samples were centrifuged and extracted prior to analysis. Samples collected in polystyrene tubes gave the same results as samples collected in glass. Storage at room temperature for 1-6 months did not affect results. Freezing introduced a constant negative offset. Stimulants to saliva flow including lemon juice and sugared gum skewed results, as did coffee or milk, although these effects varied widely between individuals.

Lo MS, Ng ML, Azmy BS, Khalid BA. Clinical applications of salivary cortisol measurements. *Sing Med J* 1992;33:170.

The circadian variation of cortisol in plasma (total cortisol) and saliva was measured in 108 normal individuals. The correlation coefficient for cortisol in the two matrices was 0.81. Comparison was also made between salivary and plasma cortisol levels in normal pregnant females, hyperthyroid patients, hypertensive patients and diabetics. The marked elevations in total plasma cortisol in these instances were not observed with salivary cortisol. The authors conclude that salivary cortisol is a better measure of adrenal status than plasma.

Lu YC, Chatterton RT, Vogelsong KM, May LK. Direct radioimmunoassay of progesterone in saliva. *J Immunoassay* 1997;18:149-163.

This study looked at various aspects of a salivary progesterone assay. The influence of the composition of the specimen collection tubes, and the composition of the analytical standards on final results was studied. Progesterone was found to adsorb on to the walls of some types of collection tubes, and standards made up in stripped saliva gave more accurate results than standards made up in a buffer. Daily salivary progesterone levels were measured in 10 women throughout the menstrual cycle, and the expected luteal phase increase was seen. Finally, matched serum and saliva specimens were collected from 48 women in the luteal phase of their cycle, and the correlation coefficient between the two sample types was found to be r=0.75.

McGregor JA, Hastings C, Roberts T, Barrett J. Diurnal variation in saliva estriol level during pregnancy: a pilot study. *Am J Obstet Gynecol* 1999; 180:S223-225.

The circadian variation of estriol level in saliva was studied in 14 pregnant women. A marked nocturnal surge in estriol occurred, with a peak between 2 and 4 a.m. These findings agree with other human and animal research on plasma estriol levels. The study demonstrates that salivary estriol correlates to plasma estriol. The authors conclude that if salivary estriol is measured for pregnancy screening purposes, samples should be acquired during daylight hours to avoid false positives.

McGregor JA, Jackson GM, Lachelin GC, Goodwin TM, Artal R, Hastings C, Dullien V. Salivary estriol as risk assessment for preterm labor: a prospective trial. *Am J Obstet Gynecol* 1995;173:1337-1342.

Serial salivary estriol monitoring in pregnancy was shown to be a better predictor of pre term labor and delivery compared to conventional risk assessment based on history. When a threshold of 2300 pg/ml was used, salivary estriol correctly predicted the occurrence of pre term labor in 77% of cases versus 37% for clinical risk score. The ability of salivary estriol to predict pre term delivery was lower (50%) but still better than risk score prediction (33%). The authors conclude, "Serial collection and measurement of salivary estriol was easy to perform and relatively effective as a means to identify women at heightened risk of pre term labor and delivery."

Meulenberg PM, Hofman JA. Salivary progesterone excellently reflects free and total progesterone in plasma during pregnancy. *Clin Chem* 1989;35:168-172.

Salivary progesterone was compared to free plasma progesterone (via equilibrium dialysis) and total serum progesterone in 36 pregnant women, sampled four times throughout pregnancy. Overall, salivary progesterone was well correlated to both free (r=0.88) and total serum progesterone (r+0.9), although salivary progesterone was on average 50% of free progesterone in serum. The authors felt that centrifugation of saliva prior to analysis may have sequestered a fraction of the progesterone in saliva. Both free serum progesterone and salivary progesterone represented 0.5-1% of total serum progesterone throughout pregnancy. In the postpartum period, binding of progesterone in serum decreased markedly (% free progesterone increased to 12% from 1%), and overall, levels of progesterone fell drastically. The authors conclude, "Despite the dramatic increase in concentrations of total progesterone and binding proteins in plasma during pregnancy, we found highly significant correlations between total and free progesterone in plasma and salivary progesterone in the group as a whole as well as individuals."

O'Leary P, Feddema P, Chan K, Taranto M, Smith M, Evans S. Salivary, but not serum or urinary levels of progesterone are elevated after topical application of progesterone cream to pre and postmenopausal women. *Clin Endocrinol* 2000;53:615-620.

This study measures the response of serum, salivary and urine progesterone and progesterone metabolites in premenopausal (n=6) and postmenopausal (n=6) women after a single application of a cream containing 64 mg of micronized progesterone. Serum levels rose marginally after cream application. Urine progesterone metabolites did not change. Saliva progesterone levels increase substantially within the first 3 hours of application. There was an approximately 7-fold greater increase in salivary progesterone levels in premenopausal women compared to postmenopausal women. On this basis, the authors conclude that no useful relationship between saliva progesterone levels and transdermal progesterone dose exists. This disparity between pre and postmenopausal transdermal progesterone levels has not been seen at ZRT Laboratory. Measurements taken after several cycles of progesterone use (2-3 weeks per cycle) might have been more relevant, giving postmenopausal women time to adapt to higher progesterone exposure.

Petsos P, Ratcliffe WA, Heath DF, Anderson DC. Comparison of blood spot, salivary and serum progesterone assays in the normal menstrual cycle. *Clin Endocrin* 1986;24:31-38.

This 1986 study compares serum, blood spot and salivary progesterone levels in 6 patients. Salivary progesterone displays the expected luteal phase increase and tracks serum progesterone well. Salivary levels correlated well (r=0.89) with serum. Despite the low sensitivity (detection limit 3000 pg/ml) and high CV (12-14%), this study demonstrates the congruence of saliva and serum progesterone measurements.

Quissell D. Steroid hormone analysis in human saliva. *Ann N Y Acad Sci.* 1993;694:143-145.

In this very brief overview of salivary steroid hormone analysis, the author mentions several possible pitfalls to analysis including: metabolization of hormones by cells of the salivary gland or oral flora, contamination of saliva by plasma from traumatized oral tissue or gingival crevicular fluid. Nevertheless, the author concludes,

"Saliva collection has provided the medical and research community with an excellent medium for the monitoring of plasma steroid levels."

Raff H, Raff JL, Findling JW. Late-night salivary cortisol as a screening test for Cushing's Syndrome. *J Clin Endocrinol Metab* 1998;83:2681-2686.

Salivary cortisol levels were studied in 73 normal individuals and 78 patients suspected of having Cushing's Syndrome. Patients with spontaneous Cushing's Syndrome were found to have a markedly elevated late-night salivary cortisol, and could be identified with a sensitivity of 97%. The authors conclude, "the measurement of late-night salivary cortisol is a simple, convenient, and reliable way to screen patients for Cushing's Syndrome."

Read GF. Status report on measurement of salivary estrogens and androgens. *Ann NY Acad Sci* 1993:146-160.

This paper reviews the status of salivary hormone testing. Some of the tentative conclusions have since been validated. This paper is primarily of historical interest.

Read G, Fahmy D, Wilson D, Griffiths K. A new approach for breast cancer research, assays for steroids in saliva. *Chronobiology International*1984, Vol. 1, No. 2, 159-165 .

This paper outlines studies validating some of the basic analytical characteristics of salivary steroid hormone assays. Levels of 17-hydroxyprogesterone and cortisol in mixed saliva correlated well (r= 0.98) with fluid collected directly from the parotid duct outlet. Serial simultaneous measurements of 17-hydroxyprogesterone in plasma, saliva and parotid fluid correlated well and displayed circadian variation. Levels of 17-hydroxyprogesterone and cortisol were equal in unstimulated and stimulated saliva samples. Plasma and salivary progesterone levels correlated well over a menstrual cycle, with salivary progesterone exhibiting the expected luteal phase increase. Women with suspected luteal phase deficiency were seen to have low or erratic levels of salivary progesterone.

Riad-Fahmy D, Read GF, Walker RF. Salivary steroid assays for assessing variation in endocrine activity. *J Steroid Biochem* 1983;19:265-272.

The correlation between plasma and saliva hormone levels in a variety of situations are presented in this paper. Plasma and salivary cortisol levels after an injection of ACTH in a normal subject, measured at 15 minute intervals were well-correlated. Cortisol measurements in saliva and plasma were also acquired every 15 minutes over a 12 hour period in 3 individuals, and again the values were very well correlated. Other data validating salivary hormone assay are also presented, including serial measurements of salivary testosterone levels illustrating the expected circadian variation over 12 hours, and serial salivary progesterone and estradiol measurements over the course of menstrual cycles, once again demonstrating expected variation. The authors note, "Studies like these illustrate the usefulness of salivary sampling regimens for monitoring short term changes in secretory activity. Since these samples unlike plasma, are easily collected by stress-free, non-invasive techniques, volunteers are more readily recruited, and undue disturbance of endocrine systems is avoided."

Ruutiainen K, Sannikka E, Santti R, Erkkola R, Adlercreutz H. Salivary testosterone in hirsutism:correlations with serum testosterone and the degree of hair growth. *J Clin Endocrinol Metab* 1987;64:1015-1020.

Testosterone was measured in saliva and serum samples in 53 females attending a hirsutism clinic. Testosterone in saliva was significantly correlated (r=0.41) to facial hirsutism whereas serum free testosterone was not correlated. The authors conclude," On the basis of the results, salivary testosterone seems to relate to the bioavailable fraction of the hormone and thus appears to be an optimal method for studying hirsute females".

Sannikka E, Terho P, Suominen J, Santti R. Testosterone concentrations in human seminal plasma and saliva and its correlation with non-protein-bound and total testosterone levels in serum. *Int J Andrology* 1983;6:319-330.

This is an early paper on salivary hormone analysis. Salivary testosterone in males was shown to be independent of saliva flow-rate (correlation between testosterone concentration in stimulated and unstimulated saliva samples was 0.96.), and whole saliva values correlated well (r=0.86) with saliva collected directly from the parotid duct. The correlation coefficient for free serum testosterone on salivary testosterone was 0.75. The salivary testosterone level correlated well with Tanner stage in adolescent boys. The authors conclude, "Determination of testosterone in saliva could thus provide a convenient and accurate index of the non-protein-bound concentration of testosterone in serum i.e. the availability of hormone to tissues."

Tschop M, Behre HM, Nieschlag E, Dressendorfer RA, Strasburger CJ. A time-resolved fluorescence immunoassay for the measurement of testosterone in saliva: monitoring of testosterone replacement therapy with testosterone buciclate. *Clin Chem Lab Med* 1998;36:223-230.

In this paper, the treatment of male hypogonadism via testosterone replacement was monitored via salivary measurements. Parallel serum and saliva samples were taken at increasing intervals after a single injection of testosterone buciclate, for a total of 16 weeks. The concentration versus time profiles for serum androgens (total testosterone + total DHT) and saliva testosterone were very similar. A weak, but significant correlation between total serum androgens and salivary testosterone (r=0.22) was seen, but no details on the timing of acquisition of saliva and blood samples were provided. Samples acquired at different times of the day would not be expected to correlate for a hormone such as testosterone for which significant circadian variation is seen. The authors conclude, "The time resolved fluorescence immunoassay for salivary testosterone provides a useful tool for monitoring androgen status in men and women, and is well suited for the follow up of testosterone replacement therapy on an outpatient basis."

Vining RF, McGinley RA, Symons RG. Hormones in saliva: mode of entry and consequent implications for clinical interpretation. *Clin Chem* 1983;29:1752-1756.

This is a landmark paper for salivary hormone analysis in which measurements of non-protein bound, unconjugated estriol and DHEA in serum are compared to "salivary estriol" and "salivary DHEA". Direct numerical agreement between the two matrices indicates that salivary hormone levels represent the non-protein bound, unconjugated, or bioavailable hormone. Consideration of the anatomy of the salivary gland, along with solubility considerations, and comparison of the concentration of conjugated hormone in saliva and serum allow the following conclusions to be drawn: Unconjugated steroids make their way into saliva by partitioning between the membranes of the acinar cells and saliva. Unconjugated steroids are largely excluded from saliva since they primarily gain entry by passage through acinar cell tight junctions. Because the concentration of conjugated estriol in serum is roughly ten times that of unconjugated estriol however, the amounts of conjugated and unconjugated estriol in saliva are roughly equal despite their different mechanisms of transport into saliva.

Worthman CM, Stallings JF, Hofman LF. Sensitive salivary estradiol assay for monitoring ovarian function. *Clin Chem* 1990;36:1769-1773.

A method for salivary estradiol assay is discussed in this paper. Samples were obtained from 15 normally-cycling women at various times in their cycles, and the expected pre-ovulatory peak was readily detected. Matched serum and saliva specimens were assayed in another group of women undergoing ovulation induction, and a correlation coefficient r=0.76 was generated. The authors conclude that, "monitoring of estradiol concentrations in saliva may provide a useful diagnostic tool that allows better resolution of some clinical problems than do values for serum alone."

Safety and Efficay of Transdermal Delivery of Hormones

Sitruk-Ware R. Transdermal delivery of steroids. *Contraception* 1989; 39(1): 1-20.

This review summarizes the advantages of delivering steroids through the skin, as well as reviews skin biology. The authors make a strong case for the choice of transdermal delivery of hormones (especially estrogen, progesterone, and testosterone) for both male and female patients with respect to safety, efficacy, and ease of use and predict this delivery method to make a significant impact on the quality of care for both male and female patients.*

Estrogens
Oral Versus Transdermal

Canonico M, Plu-Bureau G, Lowe GD, Scarabin PY. Hormone replacement therapy and risk of venous thromboembolism in post-menopausal women: systematic review and meta-analysis. *BMJ* 2008;336(7655):1227-31.

This meta-analysis of 17 studies of postmenopausal women found that those using oral estrogens had an increased risk of thromboembolism compared with those using transdermal estrogens, particularly during the first year of treatment. Even in women with pre-existing risk factors for thromboembolism, transdermal estrogen use did not confer additional risk.

Gillson GR, Zava DT. A perspective on HRT for women: picking up the pieces after the Women's Health Initiative trial - Part 1. *Int J Pharm Compounding* 2003;7(4):250-6.

This article discusses some fundamental aspects of safer hormone replacement therapy that may have been overlooked in the *debate surrounding bioidentical versus synthetic hormones: Oral delivery of hormones is not optimal; application of hormones to the skin (transdermal application) has many important advantages; and synthetic progestins are not acceptable as a substitute for natural progesterone. The evidence for and principles behind these factors are presented.**

Gillson GR, Zava DT. A perspective on HRT for women: picking up the pieces after the Women's Health Initiative trial - Part 2. *Int J Pharm Compounding* 2003;7(5):330-8.

The authors review clinical evidence for the benefits of bioidentical progesterone over synthetic progestins. While both protect the uterine lining from proliferation caused by estrogens, progesterone has beneficial effects on cardiovascular health. The synergy between progesterone and estradiol, each "turning on" the other's receptors, has the added benefit of allowing the estradiol dosage to be reduced. Oral and transdermal dosing of bioidentical progesterone are discussed.*

L'Hermite M, Simoncini T, Fuller S, Genazzani AR., Could transdermal estradiol + progesterone be a safer postmenopausal HRT? A review. *Maturitas* 2008;60(3-4):185-201.

This detailed review examines the way different types of hormone replacement therapy (HRT) affect the cardiovascular system, the brain, and the risk of breast cancer. It discusses the research that shows that non-oral estrogens have more favorable cardiovascular effects, such as improved blood pressure control and lower risk of thrombosis. It discusses the benefits of using natural progesterone rather than synthetic progestins in association with estrogens in HRT. Natural progesterone has a beneficial effect on blood vessels and the brain, and confers less or even no risk of breast cancer, compared with synthetic progestins.*

Micheline CC et al., Bioidentical estradiol cream is more effective in managing weight and insulin sensitivity than capsule form: *Fertil Steril.* 2006 Dec;86(6)1669.

Scarabin PY, Alhenc-Gelas M, Plu-Bureau G, Taisne P, Agher R, Aiach M., Effects of oral and transdermal estrogen/progesterone regimens on blood coagulation and fibrinolysis in postmenopausal women. A randomized controlled trial. *Arterioscler Thromb Vasc Biol* 1997; 17(11): 3071-8.

Oral hormone replacement therapy postmenopausally has been associated with an increased risk of stoke due to thromboembolism. This randomized, placebo-controlled study evaluated the differing effects of oral and transdermal estrogen/progesterone therapy or placebo on hemostasis. Oral, but not transdermal therapy was seen to increase the susceptibility of clotting in healthy post-menopausal women 45-64 years. The authors concluded that route of administration of hormones can affect the incidence of clotting, with oral hormone replacement increasing risk, and transdermal hormone replacement demonstrating no negative effect on clotting.*

Scarabin PY, et al. Effects of oral and transdermal estrogen/progesterone regimens on blood coagulation and fibrinolysis in postmenopausal women. A randomized, controlled trial. *Arterioscler Thromb Vasc Biol.* 1997;17(11):3071-3078.

Hyperviscosity is another important risk factor for cardiovascular disease. Studies comparing oral and transdermal delivery routes of hormones found that transdermal estradiol had no detrimental effects on coagulation and no observed risk for venous thromboembolism. In contrast, studies have documented increased risk for venous thromboembolic events (VTE) with oral CEE.*

Zegura B, Keber I, Sebestjen M, Koenig W. Double blind, randomized study of estradiol replacement therapy on markers of inflammation, coagulation and fibrinolysis. *Atherosclerosis.* 2003 May;168(1):123-9.

It has been established that Estrogen replacement therapy (ERT) is associated with increased cardiovascular risk in the first year after initiation of ERT. This study compared the effects of oral and transdermal estradiol (E2) replacement therapy on markers of inflammation, coagulation and fibrinolysis in a randomized double-blind trial over a period of 28 weeks. Forty-three healthy women were randomized 6 weeks after surgically induced menopause to receive treatment with either oral or transdermal E2 over a period of 28 weeks. At baseline and after 28 weeks, levels of serum lipids and lipoproteins, and markers of coagulation, fibrinolysis and inflammation were determined. Oral estrogen shortened clot time, both oral and transdermal estrogen reduced fibrinogen. Oral estrogen increased CRP while transdermal did not. Oral estrogen improved lipid profile while transdermal estrogen had a less profound effect on lipids and both forms significantly reduced fasting glucose. Oral E2 was associated with a pro-inflammatory response. There was no influence of transdermal E2 on markers of coagulation activation, fibrinolysis and inflammation, but it decreased fibrinogen levels significantly.

Progesterone
Transdermal versus Oral Delivery

de Ziegler D, Fanchin R. Progesterone and progestins: applications in gynecology. *Steroids* 2000;65(10-11):671-9.

*This paper reviews the use of a transvaginal progesterone gel as a viable option to other routes of application of natural progesterone (intramuscular, oral micronized), and offered it as a viable option to synthetic progestins given the low incidence of side effects noted in existing studies.**

O'Leary P, Feddema P, Chan K, Taranto M, Smith M, Evans S. Salivary, but not serum or urinary levels of progesterone are elevated after topical application of progesterone cream to pre-and postmenopausal women. *Clin Endocrinol* (Oxf) 2000;53(5):615-20.

Absorption of progesterone as provided in a topical prepara-tion of "natural" progesterone cream to 6 premenopausal and 6 postmenopausal women was demonstrated via salivary hormone levels. Salivary progesterone concentrations reached their peak 1-4 hrs after application. A five-fold increase in mean levels was seen in the premenopausal group. Serum progesterone levels were not significantly different from baseline in either group, and serum progesterone was not seen as an effective measure of absorption of topically applied progesterone. *

CHAPTER 5

Vitamin E
Painful Periods

Rasgon NL, Yargin KN. Vitamin E for the treatment of dysmenor-rhea. *BJOG*. 2005 Aug;112(8):1164.

N-Acetyl-Cysteine
Androgen Reduction

Fulghesu AM, Ciampelli M, Muzj G, Belosi C, Selvaggi L, Ayala GF, Lanzone A. N-acetyl-cysteine treatment improves insulin sensi-tivity in women with polycystic ovary syndrome. *Fertil Steril* 2002 Jun;77(6):1128-35

NAC may be a new treatment for the improvement of insulin cir-culating levels and insulin sensitivity in hyperinsulinemic patients with polycystic ovary syndrome.

Elevated Cortisol
Weight Gain

Epel ES, McEwen B, Seeman T, et al. Stress and body shape: Stress-induced cortisol secretion is consistently greater among women with central fat. *Psychosomatic Med.* 2000 Sept;62(5):623-32.

Gluck ME, Geliebter A, Lorence M. Cortisol stress response is positively correlated with central obesity in obese women with binge eating disorder (BED) before and after cognitive-behavioral treatment. Ann NY *Acad Sci.* 2004 Dec;1032:202-7.

The researchers found a positive correlation between high stress and cortisol levels and central obesity, noting, "hyperactive HPA axis due to stress raises cortisol, which may contribute to binge eating and abdominal obesity."

Chronic Stress
Cancer

van der Pompe G, Antoni MH, Heijnen CJ. Elevated basal cortisol levels and attenuated ACTH and cortisol responses to a behavioral challenge in women with metastatic breast cancer. *Psychoneuroendocrinology.* 1996 May;21(4):361-74.

Reiche EM, Nunes SO, Morimoto HK. Stress, depression, the immune system, and cancer. *Lancet Oncol.* 2004 Oct;5(10):617-25.

Chronic Stress
Hypertension

Ohlin B, Nilsson PM, Nilsson JA, Berglund G. Chronic psychosocial stress predicts long-term cardiovascular morbidity and mortality in middle-aged men. *Eur Heart J.* 2004 May;25(10):867-73.

Elevated Cortisol
Cognitive Decline

Gold PW, Drevets WC, Charney DS. New insights into the role of cortisol and the glucocorticoid receptor in severe depression. *Biol Psychiatry*. 2002 Sep 1;52(5):381-5.

Researchers have found that cortisol can affect mood and behavior, and disrupt memory and recall. Cortisol levels are directly related to the degree of cognitive impairment in people with Alzheimer's disease. These patients also had much lower levels of DHEA sulfate (DHEA-S), and therefore a dramatically higher cortisol- DHEA-S ratio than individuals without Alzheimer's.

Lupien S, Lecours AR, Lussoer I, Schwartz G, Nair NP, Meaney M. Basal cortisol levels and cognitive deficits in human aging. *J Neurosci*. 1994 May;14(5 Pt 1):2893-903.

Murialdo G, Barreca A, Nobili F, et al. Relationships between cortisol, dehydroepiandrosterone sulfate and insulin-like growth factor-I system in dementia. *J Endocrinol Invest*. 2001 Mar;24(3):139-46.

A four-year longitudinal study found a significant relationship between increasing cortisol levels and the impairment of explicit memory and selective attention performance in otherwise healthy individuals.

Pomara N, Greenberg WM, Branford MD, Doraiswamy PM. Therapeutic implications of HPA axis abnormalities in Alzheimer's disease: review and update. *Psychopharmacol Bull*. 2003;37(2):120-34.

Excessive cortisol levels have neurotoxic effects on the hippocampus, resulting in atrophy and memory impairment.

Cortisol Reduction
Phosphatidylserine

Fahey TD, Pearl MS. The hormonal and perceptive effects of phosphatidylserine administration during two weeks of resistive exercise-induced overtraining. *Biol Sport.* 1998;15:135-144.

Hellhammer J, Fries E, Buss C, et al. Effects of soy lecithin phosphatidic acid and phosphatidylserine complex (PAS) on the endocrine and psychological responses to mental stress. *Stress.* 2004 Jun;7(2):119-26.

Kidd, P. "Phosphatidylserine: A Remarkable Brain Cell Nutrient." Decatur, IL: Lucas Meyer, Inc. 1997.

Monteleone P, Maj M, Beinat L, Natale M, Kemali D. Blunting by chronic phosphatidylserine administration of the stress-induced activation of the hypothalamo-pituitary-adrenal axis in healthy men. *Eur J Clin Pharmacol.* 1992;42(4):385-8.

Monteleone P, Beinat L, Tanzillo C, Maj M, Kemali D. Effects of phosphatidylserine on the neuroendocrine response to physical stress in humans. *Neuroendocrinology.* 1990 Sep;52(3):243-8.

Cortisol Reduction
Vitamin C

Brody S, Preut R, Schommer K, Schurmeyer TH. A randomized controlled trial of high dose ascorbic acid for reduction of blood pressure, cortisol, and subjective responses to psychological stress. *Psychopharmacology* (Berl). 2002 Jan;159(3):319-24.

Peters EM, Anderson R, Nieman DC, Fickl H, Jogessar V. Vitamin C supplementation attenuates the increases in circulating cortisol, adrenaline and anti-inflammatory polypeptides following ultramarathon running. *Int J Sports Med.* 2001 Oct;22(7):537-43.

Cortisol Reduction
Fish Oil

Delarue J, Matzinger O, Binnert C, Schneeiter P, Chiolero P, Tappy L. Fish oil prevents the adrenal activation elicited by mental stress in healthy men. *Diabetes Metab.* 2003 Jun;29(3):289-95.

Cortisol Reduction
Relora

LaValle, J. and Hawkins, E. "Relora.The Natural Breakthrough to Losing Stress-Related Fat and Wrinkles." North Bergen, NJ: Basic Health Publications; 2003:16.

Cortisol Reduction
Theanine

Juneja LR, Chu D-C, Okubo T, et al. L-theanine a unique amino acid of green tea and its relaxation effect in humans. *Trends Food Sci Tech* 1999; 10:199-204.

Kimura K, Ozeki M, Juneja LR, Ohira H. L-Theanine reduces psychological and physiological stress responses. *Biol Psychol.* 2007 Jan;74(1):39-45.

Cortisol Reduction
Ginkgo

Jezova D, Duncko R, Lassanova M, Kriska M, Moncek F. Reduction of rise in blood pressure and cortisol release during stress by ginkgo biloba extract (EGB 761) in healthy volunteers. *J Physiol Pharmacol.* 2002 Sep;53(3):337-48.

Herbs
Stress Reduction

Kelly GS. Rhodiola rosea: a possible plant adaptogen. *Altern Med Rev.* 2001 Jun;6(3):293-302.

Kelly GS. Nutritional and botanical interventions to assist with the adaptation to stress. *Altern Med Rev.* 1999 Aug;4(4):249-65.

Kelly GS. Nutritional and botanical interventions to assist with the adaptation to stress. *Altern Med Rev.* 1999 Aug;4(4):249-65.

Kelly GS. Rhodiola rosea: a possible plant adaptogen. *Altern Med Rev.* 2001 Jun;6(3):293-302.

Nocerino E, Amato M, Izzo AA. The aphrodisiac and adaptogenic properties of ginseng. *Fitoterapia.* 2000 Aug;71 Suppl 1:S1-5.

Adrenal Fatigue

Wilson, J.," Adrenal Fatigue – The 21st Century Stress Syndrome". 2001; Ptealuma, Ca: Smart Publications.

Insulin Resistance

Sears, B., "The Omega Rx Zone: The Miracle of the New High-Dose Fish Oil". 2001; New York, NY: HarperCollins Publishers Inc.

Insulin Resistance
Chromium

Anderson RA, Cheng N, Bryden NA, et al. Elevated intakes of supplemental chromium improve glucose and insulin variables in individuals with type 2 diabetes. *Diabetes.* 1997 Nov;46(11):1786-91.

Bahijri SM, Mufti AM. Beneficial effects of chromium in people with type 2 diabetes, and urinary chromium response to glucose load as a possible indicator of status. *Biol Trace Elem Res.* 2002 Feb;85(2):97-109.

Bahijiri SM, Mira SA, Mufti AM, Ajabnoor MA. The effects of inorganic chromium and brewer's yeast supplementation on glucose tolerance, serum lipids and drug dosage in individuals with type 2 diabetes. *Saudi Med J.* 2000 Sep;21(9):831-7.

Wilson BE, Gondy A. Effects of chromium supplementation on fasting insulin levels and lipid parameters in healthy, non-obese young subjects. *Diabetes Res Clin Pract.* 1995 Jun;28(3):179-84.

Insulin Resistance
Vanadium

McNeill, J. Enhanced in vivo sensitivity of vanadyl-treated diabetic rats to insulin. *Canadian Journal of Physiology and Pharmacology* 1996. 68 (4):486-91.

Poucheret P, Verma S, Grynpas M, McNeill J. Vanadium and dia-betes. *Mol Cell Biochem* 1998;188(102):73-80.

Insulin Resistance
Cinnamon

Anderson RA, Broadhurst CL, Polansky MM et al. Isolation and characterization of polyphenol type-A polymers from cinnamon with insulin-like biological activity. *J Agric Food Chem.* 2004 Jan 14;52(1):65-70.

Imparl-Radosevich J, Deas S, Polansky MM, et al. Regulation of PTP-1 and insulin receptor kinase by fractions from cinnamon: implications for cinnamon regulation of insulin signalling. *Horm Res.* 1998 Sep;50(3):177-82.

Jarvill-Taylor KJ, Anderson RA, Graves DJ. A hydroxychalcone derived from cinnamon functions as a mimetic for insulin in 3T3-L1 adipocytes. *J Am Coll Nutr.* 2001 Aug;20(4):327-36.

Khan A, Safdar M, Ali Khan MM, Khattak KN, Anderson RA. Cinnamon improves glucose and lipids of people with type 2 diabetes. *Diabetes Care.* 2003 Dec;26(12):3215-8.

Kim SH, Hyun SH, Choung SY. Anti-diabetic effect of cinnamon extract on blood glucose in db/db mice. *J Ethnopharmacol.* 2006 Mar 8;104(1-2):119-23.

Qin B, Nagasaki M, Ren M, et al. Cinnamon extract prevents the insulin resistance induced by a high-fructose diet. *Horm Metab Res.* 2004 Feb;36(2):119-25.

Insulin Resistance
Goat's Rue

Petricic J, Kalodera Z. Galegin in the goats rue herb: its toxicity, antidiabetic activity and content determination. *Acta Pharm Jugosl.* 1982; 32(3):219-23.

Insulin Resistance
Alpha Lipoic Acid

Jacob S, Streeper RS, Fogt DL, et al. The antioxidant alpha-lipoic acid enhances insulin-stimulated glucose metabolism in insulin-resistant rat skeletal muscle. *Diabetes.* 1996 Aug;45(8):1024-9.

Insulin Resistance
Carnitine

Crayhon R. "The Carnitine Miracle." New York: M. Evans; 1999.

Insulin Resistance
Coenzyme Q10

McCarty MF. Can correction of sub-optimal coenzyme Q status improve beta-cell func- tion in type II diabetics? *Med Hypotheses.* 1999 May;52(5):397-400.

Insulin Resistance
Coffee Berry

Johnston KL, Clifford MN, Morgan LM. Coffee acutely modifies gastrointestinal hormone secretion and glucose tolerance in humans: glycemic effects of chlorogenic acid and caffeine. *Am J Clin Nutr.* 2003 Oct;78(4):728-33.

McCarty MF. A chlorogenic acid-induced increase in GLP-1 pro- duction may mediate the impact of heavy coffee consumption on diabetes risk. *Med Hypotheses.* 2005;64(4):848-53.

Rodriguez de Sotillo DV, Hadley M. Chlorogenic acid modi- fies plasma and liver concentrations of: cholesterol, triacylglyc- erol, and minerals in (fa/fa) Zucker rats. *J Nutr Biochem.* 2002 Dec;13(12):717-26.

Insulin Resistance
Essential Fatty Acids

Delarue J, LeFoll C, Corporeau C, Lucas D. N-3 long chain polyun- saturated fatty acids: a nutritional tool to prevent insulin resistance associated to type 2 diabetes and obesity? *Reprod Nutr Dev.* 2004 May;44(3):289-99.

Ferre P. The biology of peroxisome proliferator-activated receptors: relationship with lipid metabolism and insulin sensitivity. *Diabetes.* 2004 Feb;53 Suppl 1S43-S50.

Insulin Resistance
Magnesium

Murray MT. "Encyclopedia of Nutritional Supplements." Rocklin, CA: Prima Publishing; 1996.

Thyroid

Thyroid Deficiency

Colin M Dayan, Ponnusamy Saravanan, Graham Bayly Whose normal thyroid function is better—yours or mine? Commentary *The Lancet* 2002 Aug 03; 360 (9330): 353.

Michalopoulou G, Alevizaki M, Piperingos G, et al. High serum cholesterol levels in persons with "high-normal" TSH levels: should one extend the definition of subclinical hypothyroidism? *Eur J Endocrinol* 1998; 138: 141-45.

Vanderpump MP, Tunbridge WM, French JM, Appleton D, Bates D, Clark F, Grimley Evans J, Hasan DM, Rodgers H, Tunbridge F, et al. The incidence of thyroid disorders in the community: a twenty-year follow-up of the Whickham Survey. *Clin Endocrinol* (Oxf) 1995 Jul;43(1):55-68

Thyroid Combination Therapy

Héctor F. Escobar-Morreale, José I. Botella-Carretero, Francisco Escobar del Rey and Gabriella Morreale de Escobar. Treatment of Hypothyroidism with Combinations of Levothyroxine plus Liothyronine *The Journal of Clinical Endocrinology & Metabolism* Vol. 90, No. 8 4946-4954.

CHAPTER 6

PMS
Calcium and Vitamin D

Bertone-Johnson ER, Hankinson SE, Bendich A, Johnson SR, Willett WC, Manson JE. Calcium and vitamin D intake and risk of incident premenstrual syndrome. *Arch Intern Med.* 2005 Jun 13;165(11):1246-52.

Thys-Jacobs S. Micronutrients and the premenstrual syndrome: The case for calcium. *J Am Coll Nutr.* 2000 Apr;19(2):220–7.

Thys-Jacobs S, Starkey P, et al. Calcium carbonate and the premenstrual syndrome: Effects on premenstrual and menstrual symptoms. Premenstrual Syndrome Study Group. *Am J Obstet Gynecol.* 1998 Aug;179(2):444–52.

Thys-Jacobs S. Alleviation of migraines with therapeutic vitamin D and calcium. *Headache.* 1994 Nov-Dec;34(10):590-2.

PMS
Magnesium

Abraham GE, Lubran MM. Serum and red cell magnesium levels in patients with premenstrual tension. *Am J Clin Nutr.* 1981 Nov;34(11):2364–6.

Facchinetti F, Borella P, et al. Oral magnesium successfully relieves premenstrual mood changes. *Obstet Gynecol.* 1991 Aug;78(2):177–81.

Muneyyirci-Delale O, Nacharaju VL, Dalloul M, et. al, Serum ionized magnesium and calcium in women after menopause: Inverse relation of estrogen with ionized magnesium. *Fertil Steril.* 1999;71:869-872.

Seelig, M. S., Interrelationship of magnesium and estrogen in cardiovascular and bone disorders, eclampsia, migraine and premenstrual syndrome. *J Am Coll Nutr.* 12: 4, Aug 1993,442-58.

Walker AF, De Souza MC, Vickers MF, Abeyasekera S, Collins ML, Trinca LA. Magnesium supplementation alleviates premenstrual symptoms of fluid retention. *J Womens Health.* 1998 Nov;7(9):1157-65.

PMS
Zinc

Chuong CJ, Dawson EB. Zinc and copper levels in premenstrual syndrome. *Fertil Steril.* 1994 Aug;62(2):313–20.

PMS
Viamin B6

Kendall KE, Schnurr PP. The effects of vitamin B6 supplementation on premenstrual symptoms. *Obstet Gynecol.* 1987 Aug;70(2):145–9.

Wyatt KM, Dimmock PW, et al. Efficacy of vitamin B-6 in the treatment of premenstrual syndrome: Systematic review. *BMJ.* 1999 May 22;318(7195):1375–81.

PMS
Vitamin E

London RS, Murphy L, et al. Efficacy of alpha-tocopherol in the treatment of the premenstrual syndrome. *J Reprod Med.* 1987 Jun;32(6):400–4.

PMS
Essential Fatty Acids

Brush MG, Watson SJ, et al. Abnormal essential fatty acid levels in plasma of women with premenstrual syndrome. *Am J Obstet Gynecol.* 1984 Oct 15;150(4):363–6.

Harel Z, Biro FM, et al. Supplementation with omega-3 polyunsaturated fatty acids in the management of dysmenorrhea in adolescents. *Am J Obstet Gynecol.* 1996 Apr;174(4):1335–8.

Horrobin DF. The role of essential fatty acids and prostaglandins in the premenstrual syndrome. *J Reprod Med.* 1983 Jul;28(7):465–8.

Koshikawa N, Tatsunuma T, et al. Prostaglandins and premenstrual syndrome. *Prostaglandins Leukot Essent Fatty Acids.* 1992;45(1):33–6.

Piccoli A, Modena F, et al. Reduction in urinary prostaglandin excretion in the premenstrual syndrome. *J Reprod Med.* 1993;38(12):941–4.

Sampalis F, Bunea R, et al. Evaluation of the effects of Neptune Krill Oil on the management of premenstrual syndrome and dysmenorrhea. *Altern Med Rev.* 2003 May;8(2):171–9.

PMS
Chaste Tree

Halaska M, Raus K, et al. [Treatment of cyclical mastodynia using an extract of Vitex agnus castus: Results of a double-blind comparison with a placebo]. *Ceska Gynekol.* 1998 Oct;63(5):388–92.

Schellenberg R. Treatment for the premenstrual syndrome with agnus castus fruit extract: Prospective, randomised, placebo controlled study. *BMJ.* 2001 Jan 20;322(7279):134–7.

Wuttke W, Jarry H, et al. Chaste tree (Vitex agnus-castus): Pharmacology and clinical indications. *Phytomedicine.* 2003 May;10(4):348–57.

PMS
Neurotransmitters

Clayton AH, Keller AE, et al. Exploratory study of premenstrual symptoms and serotonin variability. *Arch Womens Ment Health.* 2006 Jan;9(1):51–7.

Freeman EW, Sammel MD, et al. Premenstrual syndrome as a predictor of menopausal symptoms. *Obstet Gynecol.* 2004 May;103(5 Pt 1):960–6.

Turner EH, Loftis JM, et al. Serotonin a la carte: Supplementation with the serotonin precursor 5-hydroxytryptophan. *Pharmacol Ther.* 2006 Mar;109(3):325–38.

Rapkin A. A review of treatment of premenstrual syndrome and premenstrual dysphoric disorder. *Psychoneuroendocrinology.* 2003 Aug;28 Suppl 3:39–53.

PMS
Predictor of Menopausal Symptoms

Freeman EW, Sammel MD, et al. Premenstrual syndrome as a predictor of menopausal symptoms. *Obstet Gynecol.* 2004 May;103(5 Pt 1):960–6.

Dysmenorrhea /Menstrual Pain
Vitamin E

Ziaei S, Faghihzadeh S, Sohrabvand F, et al. A randomized placebo-controlled trial to determine the effect of vitamin E in treatment of primary dysmenorrhoea. *BJOG.* 2001;108:1181-1183.

Ziaei S, Zakeri M, Kazemnejad A, et al. A randomised controlled trial of vitamin E in the treatment of primary dysmenorrhoea. *BJOG.* 2005;112:466-469.

Dysmenorrhea /Menstrual Pain
Essential Fatty Acids

Proctor M, Farquhar C. Dysmenorrhoea. *Clin Evid.* 2002; (7):1639—53.

Deutch B. Menstrual pain in Danish women correlated with low n-3 polyunsaturated fatty acid intake. *Eur J Clin Nutr.* 1995;49:508—16.

Harel Z, Biro FM, Kottenhahn RK, et al. Supplementation with omega-3 polyunsaturated fatty acids in the management of dysmenorrhea in adolescents. *Am J Obstet Gynecol.* 1996;174:1335-1338.

Dysmenorrhea /Menstrual Pain
Magnesium

Seifert B, Wagler P, Dartsch S, et al. Magnesium—a new therapeutic alternative in primary dysmenorrhea [translated from German]. *Zentralbl Gynakol.* 1989;111:755-760.

Fontana-Klaiber H, Hogg B. The therapeutic effects of magnesium in dysmenorrhea [in German; English abstract]. *Schweiz Rundsch Med Prax.* 1990;79:491-494.

Dysmenorrhea /Menstrual Pain
Accupuncture

Helms JM. Acupuncture for the management of primary dysmenorrhea. *Obstet Gynecol.* 1987;69:51-56.

Indole- 3- Carbinol

Bradlow H. L., Sepkovic D. W., Telang N. T., Osborne M. P. Indole-3-carbinol: A novel approach to breast cancer prevention. *Ann. N.Y. Acad. Sci.* 1995;768:180-200.

Broadbent T. A., Broadbent H. S. 1–1. The chemistry and pharmacology of indole-3-carbinol (indole-3-methanol) and 3-(methoxymethyl)indole. [Part I]. *Curr. Med. Chem.* 1998a;5:337-352.

Broadbent T. A., Broadbent H. S. 1. The chemistry and pharmacology of indole-3-carbinol (indole-3-methanol) and 3-(methoxymethyl)indole. [Part II]. *Curr. Med. Chem.* 1998b;5:469-491.

Chang Y. C., Riby J., Chang G. H., Peng B. C., Firestone G., Bjeldanes L. F. Cytostatic and antiestrogenic effects of 2-(indol-3-ylmethyl)-3,3'-diindolylmethane, a major in vivo product of dietary indole-3-carbinol. *Biochem. Pharmacol.* 1999;58:825-834.

Chen I., McDougal A., Wang F., Safe S. Aryl hydrocarbon-mediated antiestrogenic and antitumorigenic activity of diindolymethane. *Carcinogenesis* 1998;19:1631-1639.

Cover C. M., Hsieh S. J., Cram E. J., Hong C., Riby J. E., Bjeldanes L. F., Firestone G. L. Indole-3-carbinol and tamoxifen cooperate to arrest the cell cycle of MCF-7 human breast cancer cells. *Cancer Res* 1999;59:1244-1251.

Cover C. M., Hsieh S. J., Tran S. H., Hallden G., Kim G. S., Bjeldanes L. F., Firestone G. L. Indole-3-carbinol inhibits the expression of cyclin-dependent kinase-6 and induces a G 1 cell cycle arrest of human breast cancer cells independent of estrogen receptor signaling. *J. Biol. Chem.* 1998;273:3838-3847.

Ge X., Fares F. A., Yannai S. Induction of apoptosis in MCF-7 cells by indol-3-carbinol is independent of p53 and bax. *Anticancer Res* 1999;19:3199-3203.

Hudson E. A., Howells L., Ball H. W., Pfeifer A. M., Manson M. M. Mechanisms of action of indole-3-carbinol as a chemopreventive agent. *Biochem. Soc. Trans.* 1998;26:S370.

Jin L., Qi M., Chen D. Z., Anderson A., Yang G. Y., Arbeit I. M., Auborn K. I. Indole-3-carbinol prevents cervical cancer in human papilloma virus type 16 (HPV16) transgenic mice. *Cancer Res* 1999;59:3991-3997.

Kojima T., Tanaka T., Mori H. Chemoprevention of spontaneous endometrial cancer in female donryu rats by indole-3-carbinol. *Cancer Res* 1994;54:1446-1449.

Meng Q., Qi M., Chen D. Z., Goldberg I., Rosen E., Auborn K., Fan S. Suppression of breast cancer invasion and migration by indole-3-carbinol: associated with up-regulation of BRCA1 and E-cadherin/catenin complexes. *J. Mol. Med.* 2000a;78:155-165.

Meng Q, Goldberg ID, Rosen EM, Fan S. Inhibitory effects of Indole-3-carbinol on invasion and migration in human breast cancer cells.*Breast Cancer Res Treat.* 2000 Sep;63(2):147-52.

Michnovicz J. J., Bradlow H. L. Induction of estradiol metabolism by dietary indole-3-carbinol in humans. *J. Natl. Cancer Inst.* 1990;82:947-949.

Niwa T., Swaneck G., Bradlow H. L. Alterations in estradiol metabolism in MCF-7 cells induced by treatment with indole-3-carbinol and related compounds. *Steroids* 1994;59:523-527.

Tiwari R. K., Guo L., Bradlow H. L., Telang N. T., Osborne M. P. Selective responsiveness of human breast cancer cells to indole-3-carbinol, a chemopreventive agent. *J. Natl. Cancer Inst.* 1994;86:126-131.

Wong G. Y., Bradlow L., Sepkovic D., Mehl S., Mailman J., Osborne M. P. Dose-ranging study of indole-3-carbinol for breast cancer prevention. *J. Cell Biochem.* 1997;28–29:111-116.

Yuan F., Chen D. Z., Liu K., Sepkovic D. W., Bradlow H. L., Auborn K. Anti-estrogenic activities of indole-3-carbinol in cervical cells: implication for prevention of cervical cancer. *Anticancer Res* 1999;19:1673-1680.

CHAPTER 7

Homocysteine

McLean RR, Jacques PF, Selhub J, et al. Homocysteine as a predictive factor for hip fracture in older persons. *N Engl J Med.* 2004;350:2042-9.

Low Testosterone

Oronzo et al. Salivary testosterone is associated with higher lumbar bone mass in premenopausal healthy women with normal levels of serum testosterone. *Eur J Epidemiology* 16: 907-912, 2000.

Slemenda et al. Sex Steroids, Bone Mass and Bone Loss. *J Clin Invest* 97: 14-21, 1996.

Strontium

Adami S. Protelos: Nonvertebral and hip antifracture efficacy in postmenopausal osteoporosis. *Bone.* 2006 Feb;38(2 Suppl 1):23–7.

Bertrand, N. The Spinal Osteoporosis Therapeutic Intervention trial. *Joint Bone Spine* Volume 71, Issue 4, July 2004, Pages 261-263.

Burlet N, Reginster JY. Strontium ranelate: The first dual acting treatment for postmenopausal osteoporosis. *Clin Orthop Relat Res.* 2006 Feb;443:55–60.

Hall, D.A. "The Aging of Connective Tissue", Academic Press, San Francisco, 1976.

Henrotin Y., Labasse A., Zheng S.X., Galais P., Tsouderos Y., Crielaard J.M., Reginster J.Y. Strontium ranelate increases cartilage matrix formation. *J Bone Miner Res*, 2001, Feb; 16(2):299-308.

Meunier, P.J., Roux, C., Seeman, E., Ortolani, S., Badurski, J.E., Spector, T.D., Cannata, J., Balogh, A., Lemmel, E.M., Pors-Nielsen, S., Rizzoli R., Genant, H.K., Reginster J.Y. The effects of strontium ranelate on the risk of vertebral fracture in women with postmenopausal osteoporosis, *N Engl J Med*, 2004, Jan 29;350(5):459-68.

Meunier, P.J., Slosman, D.O., Delmas, P.D., Sebert, J.L., Brandi, M.L., Albanese, C., Lorenc, R., Pors-Nielsen, S., De Vernejoul, M.C., Roces, A., Reginster J.Y. Strontium ranelate: dose-dependent effects in established postmenopausal vertebral osteoporosis — a 2-year randomized placebo controlled trial. *J Clin Endocrinol Metab*, May 2002; 87(5):2060-6.

Ortolani S, Vai S. Strontium ranelate: An increased bone quality leading to vertebral antifracture efficacy at all stages. *Bone.* 2006 Feb;38(2 Suppl 1):19–22.

Reginster, J.Y., Deroisy, R., Dougados, M., Jupsin, I., Colette, J., Roux, C. Prevention of early postmenopausal bone loss by strontium ranelate: the randomized, two-year, double-masked, dose-ranging, placebo-controlled PREVOS trial. *Osteoporos Int,* 2002, Dec;13(12): 925-31.

Reginster, J.Y., Bruyère, A., Sawicki, A., Roces-Varela, P, Fardellone, A. Roberts, J. Devogelaer Long-term treatment of postmenopausal osteoporosis with strontium ranelate: Results at 8 years. *Bone*,2009 Dec; Volume 45, Issue 6, Pages 1059-1064.

Ipriflavone

Affinito P; Palomba S; et al. Postmenopausal osteoporosis: therapeutic approaches *Minerva Ginecol,* Mar 49(3):109-20 1997.

Agnusdei D; Bufalino L Efficacy of ipriflavone in established osteoporosis and long-term safety. *Calcif Tissue Int*, 61 Suppl 1:S23-7 1997.

Agnusdei D; Zacchei F; et al. Metabolic and clinical effects of ipriflavone in established post-menopausal osteoporosis *Drugs Exp Clin Res*, 61 Suppl 1(1):97-104 1989.

Attila BK Overview of clinical studies with ipriflavone *Acta Pharm Hung*, 61 Suppl 1(2):223-8 1995 Nov.

Fiore CE; et al. Modification of cortical and trabecular mineral density of the femur, induced by ipriflavone therapy, Clinical results after 12 months *Clin Ter,* 61 Suppl 1(1):13-9 1995 Jan.

Gambacciani, M, et al. Ipriflavone prevents the bone mass reduction in premenopausal women treated with gonadotropin hormone-releasing hormone agonists. *Bone and Mineral*, Volume 26, Issue 1, 1994, Pages 19-26.

Gennari C; Adami S; et al. Effect of chronic treatment with ipriflavone in postmenopausal women with low bone mass. *Calcif Tissue Int*, 61 Suppl 1(Adami S):S19-22 1997.

Kakai, Yoshio, et al. Effect of Ipriflavone and Estrogen on the Differentiation and Proliferation of Osteoclast Cells, *Calcified Tissue International*, 1992 Springer-Verlag, New York.

Kitatani K; Morii H, Ipriflavone *Nippon Rinsho*, 62):1537-43 1998 Jun.

Melis, G.B., et al. Lack of any estrogenic effect of ipriflavone in postmenopausal women. *J Endocrinol Invest*, 15: 755-61, 1992.

Miyauchi, A., et al. Novel ipriflavone receptors coupled to calcium influx regulate osteoclast differentiation and function. *Endocrinology*, 13: 3544-50, 1996.

Notoya K; et al. Stimulatory effect of ipriflavone on formation of bone-like tissue in rat bone marrow stromal cell culture. *Calcif Tissue Int*, 51 Suppl 1(-AD-):S16-20 1992.

Petilli, M., et al. Interactions between ipriflavone and the estrogen receptor. *Calcif Tissue Int*, 56: 160-65,1995.

Sz´ant´o F. Experience with ipriflavone therapy in postmenopausal osteoporosis. *Orv Hetil*, 61 Suppl 1(1):2801-3 1997 Nov 2.

Bisphosphonates

Greenspan SL, Harris ST, Bone H, et al. Bisphosphonates: safety and efficacy in the treatment of prevention of osteoporosis. *Am Fam Physician*. 2000;61:2731-2736.

Liberman UA, Weiss SR, Broll J, Minne HW, Quan H, Bell NH, et al. Effect of oral alendronate on bone mineral density and the incidence of fractures in postmenopausal osteoporosis. The Alendronate Phase III Osteoporosis Treatment Study Group. *N Engl J Med* 1995;333:1437-43.

McClung M, Clemmesen B, Daifotis A, Gilchrist NL, Eisman J, Weinstein RS, et al. Alendronate prevents postmenopausal bone loss in women without osteoporosis. Alendronate Osteoporosis Prevention Study Group. *Ann Intern Med* 1998;128:253-61.

Bisphosphonates
Side Effects

Aki S, Eskiyurt N, et al. Gastrointestinal side effect profile due to the use of alendronate in the treatment of osteoporosis. *Yonsei Med J.* 2003 Dec;44(6):961–7.

Bisphosphonates
Eye Problems

Fraunfelder FW, Fraunfelder FT. Adverse ocular drug reactions recently identified by the National Registry of Drug Induced Ocular Side Effects. *Ophthalmology.* 2004 Jul;111(7):1275–9.

Fraunfelder FW, Fraunfelder FT, et al. Scleritis and other ocular side effects associated with pamidronate disodium. *Am J Opthalmol.* 2003 Feb;135(2):219–21.

Bisphosphonates
Fracture Risk

Cheung, R., et al. 2007. Sequential nontraumatic femoral shaft fractures in a patient on long-term alendronate. *Hong Kong Med. J., 13* (6), 485–489.

McClung, M., et al. 2004. Prevention of postmenopausal bone loss: Six-year results from the Early Postmenopausal Intervention Cohort (EPIC) study. *J. Clin. Endocrinol. Metab., 89* (10), 4879–4885.

Neviaser, A., et al. 2008. Low-energy femoral shaft fractures associated with alendronate use. *J. Orthop. Trauma, 22* (5), 346–350.

Parker–Pope, Tara. 2008. Drugs to build bones may weaken them. *New York Times,* July 15, 2008.

Bisphosphonates
Bone Death in the Jaw

Fehm, T., et al. 2009. Bisphosphonate-induced osteonecrosis of the jaw (ONJ): Incidence and risk factors in patients with breast cancer and gynecological malignancies. *Gynecol. Oncol.*

Farrugia MC, Summerlin DJ, et al. Osteonecrosis of the mandible or maxilla associated with the use of new generation bisphosphonates. *Laryngoscope*. 2006 Jan;116(1):115–20.

Sedghizadeh, P., et al. 2009. Oral bisphosphonate use and th prevalence of osteonecrosis of the jaw: An institutional inquiry. *J. Am. Dent. Assoc. 140* (1), 61–66.

Bisphosphonates
Side Effects with NSAIDs

Graham DY, Malaty HM., Alendronate and naproxen are synergistic for development of gastric ulcers. *Arch Intern Med*. 2001 Jan 8;161(1):107-10.

Evista and Risk of Stokes

Barrett-Connor E et al., Effects of Raloxifene on Cardiovascular Events and Breast Cancer in Postmenopausal Women. *N Engl J Med* 2006;355:125-37.

ABOUT DONNA WHITE

Donna White, BHRT Clinical Education Consultant, works with Deborah Matthew, MD at Signature Wellness – a medical practice specializing in Bioidentical Hormone Replacement Therapy for women and men. She has written BHRT protocols and treatment plans for numerous physicians since 2001, including Dr. Dino Kanelos in Charlotte, NC, and Dr. Larry Webster and Dr. Julius Torelli in High Point, NC. She has accumulated over two hundred Continuing Education training hours at BHRT medical symposiums. She also has served as a scientific advisor and product formulator for two supplement companies.

As an educator, Donna has traveled across the U.S., training medical practitioners in how to prescribe and implement BHRT in their medical practice. She has spoken at numerous medical conferences on BHRT for physicians and compounding pharmacists. She has trained over thirty medical practices in BHRT. Donna developed a comprehensive twelve hour Continuing Education program and a six hour clinical training program to educate and train health care providers. Donna has written numerous magazine articles geared to women and has appeared on a variety of news and educational radio and television programs. She hosted the *Living Naturally* radio program for four years. Donna speaks regularly to women's groups, including Christian women's conferences and business and professional groups. In 2004 she developed The Hormone Makeover seminar and published *The Complete Hormone Makeover* DVD. She is currently sharing *The Hormone Makeover—Seven Steps to Transform Your Life with Bioidentical Hormones*, via public speaking and on her web show. She resides in Charlotte, NC, with her husband Jack and four children.

Contact Information:

Web Site
www.donnawhitehormonemakeover.com

Visit Donna on Facebook
www.facebook.com/TheDonnaWhiteHormoneMakeover

Folllow Donna on Twitter
http://twitter.com/hormonemakeover

Donna's Blog
http://hormonemakeover.blogspot.com/

DONNA WHITE SEMINARS

"A clear, concise and passionate message that can change a woman's and her family's life."
Eldred Taylor, M.D., Assistant Clinical Professor of Gynecology at Emory University and author of "Are Your Hormones Making You Sick?"

"Donna presents a very rational approach to help identify and correct hormonal imbalances with natural hormones."
David Zava, Ph.D., ZRT Laboratory, author of "What Your Doctor May Not Tell You About Breast Cancer: "

"She is a dynamic, interesting speaker who is clearly passionate about her work. Don't miss the opportunity to hear what she has to say."
George Gilson, M.D., Ph.D., Rocky Mountain Analytical Lab, Alberta, Canada, author of "Menopause: Now What?"

"White gives a valuable and clinical perspective on hormone replacement and related issues. Most clinicians need to hear what she has to teach."
James Wilson, N.D., Ph.D., D.C., author of "Adrenal Fatigue; the 21st Century Stress Syndrome."

"Donna White's knowledge of women's health and her genuine compassion is evident in her presentation of "Hormone Solutions." She provided the women in our church with simple, workable changes that could improve their physical and emotional health, while also presenting avenues for more extensive help. Donna imparts hope for hormone balance all stages of a woman's life. She showed us that natural hormone replacement has the potential to revolutionize the quality of a woman's life!"

Angie Thompson, Women's Ministry, Heritage International Ministries, Fort Mill, SC.

CPSIA information can be obtained at www.ICGtesting.com
Printed in the USA
BVOW02s1408121114

374742BV00003BA/763/P